Listening with the Whole Body

Sheila M. Frick, OTR
with
Colleen Hacker, MS, OTR

Responsible use of this material

While the authors have made great efforts to provide clear, accurate information, it is the responsibility of the reader/practitioner to evaluate the information and consult appropriate resources when considering new or unfamiliar procedures. Each practitioner is responsible for determining the appropriateness of a given intervention approach with respect to the specific individual and clinical situation. The authors, editors and the publisher cannot be held responsible for any misinterpretation or misuse of this material.

Listening with the Whole Body
© 2001 Vital Links, Madison, WI
ISBN #0-9717653-3-2

Reproducing pages from this book

Permission is granted to reproduce pages 3-76 to 3-90 for clinic or home use (not for resale). To avoid stress on your book, you may want to make a photocopy of those pages to use as your master for reproducing more.

Trademark

The term **Therapeutic Listening**™ has been trademarked to prevent confusing this approach with other sound therapy programs. While many professionals use a variety of sound therapy techniques, Therapeutic Listening refers specifically to the framework that integrates sound technology from a variety of sources with principles of occupational therapy and sensory integrative therapy in discretely applied ways. Therapeutic Listening is a trademarked term that may not be legally used in the description of any other listening program.

Editorial/ Layout Services: Eileen Richter, MPH, OTR, FAOTA
Edit/Proofing Services: Alexis Richter

About the Authors

Sheila Frick, OTR has practiced in a variety of treatment settings including hospitals, school systems, and community-based programs since graduating from Eastern Michigan University in 1980 with a degree in occupational therapy. Her interest in pediatrics and sensory processing dysfunction led to further training in sensory integration, SIPT certification, craniosacral therapy, respiratory development and treatment as well as various listening interventions including Auditory Integration Training, Listening Fitness and SAMONAS Sound Therapy. Ms. Frick's expertise in these areas has made her a popular lecturer through out the United States and abroad. She has taught core level SAMONAS with Ingo Steinbach since 1998. Training therapists to incorporate auditory intervention into a sensory integrative treatment model has become a particular goal for her.

Ms. Frick is the founder of Therapeutic Resources, a community based private practice in Madison, WI. She is the 1994 recipient of the Wisconsin Occupation Therapy Association's award of Excellence for Clinical Practice. Her publication credits include: *MORE: Integrating the Mouth with Sensory and Postural Functions; Out of the Mouths of Babes* (coauthor); many newsletter articles and an audiotape on respiration. She has been instrumental in facilitating the production of high quality, music recordings appropriate to include in Therapeutic Listening programs, e.g. *Mozart for Modulation, Baroque for Modulation, Rhythm & Rhyme, Kidz Jamz, etc.*

Colleen Hacker, MS, OTR graduated from the University of Texas Medical Branch with an undergraduate degree in Occupational Therapy in 1984. She received her master's degree with a specialization in pediatric occupational therapy from the Medical College of Virginia in 1988. Her entire occupational therapy career has been focused on pediatrics, specializing in working with children with sensory processing dysfunction. She has worked in a range of treatment environments including public schools, health departments, pediatric rehabilitation and the NICU. Since 1988, she has worked primarily in private practice settings, including 10 years at Developmental Therapy Associates, Inc. in Durham, NC before becoming clinical director of Therapeutic Resources, Inc. in Madison, WI. She is currently co-owner and clinic director of Therapeutic Associates, LLC in Madison, Wisconsin. She is trained in a variety of listening techniques including Auditory Integration Training, Listening Fitness, SAMONAS Sound Therapy and Therapeutic Listening. She collaborates with Sheila Frick on a number of teaching and professional projects.

Acknowledgments

The authors would like to thank all the therapists they have trained, who supported expansion of the model and convinced us that this book needed to be written. Thank you to the children and families who taught us so much and hopefully benefitted in return.

Thanks to Patricia Oetter, Nancy Lawton-Shirley, Steven J. Cool, Patricia Wilbarger, Mary Kawar, Ingo Steinbach and Paul Madaule for reviewing drafts and suggesting revisions, but especially for mentorship, encouragement and support to trust our clinical instincts and expand existing treatment models.

There were many who made helpful contributions that have made this book possible and who have our grateful thanks:

Tim Hamele, Ron Frick, Patricia Oetter and Alexis Richter for proofing and editing help.

Denise Neigh, Ginger Mitchell, Lori Rothman, Genevieve Jereb, Linda Lutzier, Joanne Holmes, Eileen Hamele, Lynette Burke, Molly Kaliher and Susan Richey for sharing their successes.

Jennifer Muse and Wendy Veder for assistance with the original pamphlet that grew into this book.

Josephine Moore who gave us permission to use some of her classic illustrations.

Michael (Keebler) Felknor for Figures 2-3, 2-8, 3-21 & 3-22.

Connie Hewitt and Lance Wilkinson for always being at the other end of the phone line.

Eileen Richter for her unending patience and support, for without her this book would still be a draft.

Steve Richter for countless rides to and from the airport.

Ron, Sean and Kelly Frick for sharing family time so this project could be completed.

This Book is Dedicated

To my father, Edward McLaughlin, who passed on to me the joy of learning and teaching. And to my family, Ron, Sean & Kelly, who supported this vision long before it was clear to me.

Sheila

To my parents, John and Agnes Hacker, who have supported me through every endeavor in my life. And who, like me, never imagined that my choice of OT as a career would lead to such continuously unfolding adventure.

Colleen

And to the children and their families who keep us young at heart by sustaining our ability to see the wonder in the world and our belief that all things are possible.

Sheila and Colleen

Table of Contents

Foreword

This book is an important contribution to the practice of occupational therapy. It offers another piece of the puzzle in treating clients with disorders of, or delays in sensory processing. Sheila Frick and Colleen Hacker are acute observers of behaviors and have developed their listening techniques through a constant clinical reasoning process in trying to improve client functioning. Their expansion and clinical application of the early work on listening is significant in that it places listening within the sphere of treatment for sensory modulation disorders, and it couples treatment for listening with sensory integrative occupational therapy. *Listening with the Whole Body* provides a missing link in the treatment of sensory processing deficits. Thank you Sheila and Colleen; Jean Ayres would have been proud!

Judith G. Kimball, PhD, OTR/L, FAOTA
Professor, University of New England
Author: Sensory integrative frame of reference. (1993) In
    Kramer, P. & Hinojosa, J. *Frames of Reference for Pediatric*
    Occupational Therapy. Baltimore, MD: Williams & Wilkins.

"I envision the day when Listening Training and Sound Stimulation programs will be accessible everywhere children need them; in the school, in the practitioner's office or at home. Sheila Frick's book will greatly contribute to making this dream come true. Well documented, practical and user friendly, this guide should be on the reading list of anyone interested in child development."

Paul Madaule, Director
The Listening Centre
Author: *When Listening Comes Alive.* (1993) Norval, Ontario:
    Moulin

When I first heard that Sheila Frick was developing courses on Therapeutic Listening, I knew that this would be important information for the therapists in our practice. As clinicians specializing in sensory integration, we often used music and song as part of our intervention with positive effects, but frequently problems such as auditory defensiveness and gravitational insecurity changed slowly. We were strongly interested in expanding our knowledge of sound and music to better serve our clients. We were very fortunate to sponsor one of Sheila Frick's first workshops in Therapeutic Listening. As we began to use the specially filtered music with our clients, we saw many positive results, not only in areas related to the auditory and vestibular systems, but in many areas of function.

Sheila Frick and Colleen Hacker have worked extensively using Therapeutic Listening with clients in their own practice. They have offered training courses to many therapists throughout the country and around the world with Ingo Steinbach and independently. They are now taking all of their experience to date and sharing their valuable insights with us through *Listening with the Whole Body*. This book is an excellent guide for therapists who have taken the Listening with the Whole Body course and who are now adding Therapeutic Listening to their repertoire of intervention techniques. The wealth of clinical examples and case stories beautifully illustrate the intervention principles outlined in this comprehensive book. Sheila Frick, together with Colleen Hacker, have made an excellent contribution to the field of occupational therapy, and in turn, to the many children and adults we serve.

Jane Koomar, PhD, OTR/L, FAOTA
Executive Director
Occupational Therapy Associates-Watertown, P.C.
Watertown, Massachusetts

We are physicians with a three year old daughter who has been receiving Therapeutic Listening with great success since she was eighteen months old. Sheila Frick's work is pioneering in its use of sound in combination with sensory integrative treatment techniques.

Colleen Hacker and the gifted therapists at their clinic enhance neurologic function in children with a variety of disorders, including the autism spectrum, cerebral palsy, attention deficit/hyperactivity disorder and sensory integrative disorders. A combination of auditory and other sensory stimulation activates function in cerebral areas of the brain.

In *Listening with the Whole Body*, the authors present the essential elements which provide therapists the opportunity to utilize these valuable tools. It is our hope that the anecdotal success stories in this book will inspire research into the precise causes of these disorders and guide us all in knowing which treatment is best for each child.

Karen A. Dana, MD
Gary L. Cohen, MD

Introduction

Adam

When Adam was born his mother and father were unaware of the difficulties that lay ahead for them and for Adam. Although his development seemed typical initially, around 13 months of age Adam completely stopped responding verbally to all social cues. Following lines around the family home and spinning in circles quickly became preoccupations. "At first we thought it was cute," said Jenny, Adam's mother. Soon, Adam's parents were to discover that something was seriously wrong. Adam stopped sleeping. "He would scream for hours in a very high pitched squeal. We took turns with him through the night. Sometimes I would just stand in the shower to block out the sound."

"Adam was afraid of everything," said his mother. "Whenever he saw smoke or steam or dust he would panic." Hitting and banging his head became a regular occurrence and all attempts at offering Adam comfort were fiercely resisted. "That was the hardest part," said Jenny. "There was nothing I could do." The only time Adam seemed happy to his parents was when he was alone in his darkened bedroom. During these times the light had to be turned off and no other person was allowed to enter the room.

From this early age Adam was terrified of people. When people looked at him he would quickly cover his eyes. Adam hated being touched. He demonstrated no sign of affection to any significant person in his life. He didn't appear to register pain. His mother spoke of a day when he placed his hand into a burning flame in the fire place. Initially he appeared indifferent to the blisters on his hand. When the pain of the burn eventually registered, Adam could not be comforted. Attempts to hold him led to excessive screams and panic. "All I could do was stand there and cry," said his mother. There were other times that Adam would scream until his nose bled. His mother and father felt that he was in great pain all of the time. "It just seemed really sad," said Jenny. She felt that there was much that Adam wanted to tell. "It would be like walking around all day with tape over your mouth," she said with a deep sadness. Any attempts at communica-

1

tion consisted of grunts and sounds. Eye contact was avoided. Adam was diagnosed with autism.

◆

With an early history of reflux, feeding quickly became another heartbreaking struggle for Adam and his family. Most foods seemed to be aversive to him and his appetite was extremely poor. His diet was limited to eight specific foods - they could be summed up in two categories: starch and peas.

At the age of two Adam came to the clinic for an occupational therapy evaluation. It had been a very difficult year for the family. By observing Adam and taking a sensory history it was determined that he displayed symptoms indicative of severe sensory defensiveness.

In combination with the Wilbarger Touch Pressure Protocol, a Therapeutic Listening program was implemented using modulated music.

Wearing head phones was no easy task for this sensory defensive two year old. Jenny used many strategies to familiarize Adam with the listening protocol. "I would wear them on my head while I was cooking or just around the house." she said with a smile. Playing the CD as background music also helped Adam acclimate to the music.

Within the first month significant changes in modulation occurred. His mother noted, "When Adam was screaming I would put the music on and he would begin to calm and relax. Sometimes he'd even fall asleep." Adam was beginning to sleep through the night. Babbling and eye contact were increasing. Happily, Adam had begun experimenting with expressions of affection such as cuddling, hand holding and hugging. Although still cautious, his tolerance of having others in his physical space was beginning to change. Hesitantly, he began to explore moving his body over different surfaces in the clinic space.

In three months Adam's previously terrifying relationship with the world was beginning to take on new meaning. His food repertoire increased by 10 different foods. Different textures and tactile experiences were becoming objects of interest. And to his parents' pleasure, Adam was beginning to notice other children who were playing around him. Cautiously, yet curiously he watched them play from afar. Moving in the clinic space was becoming less threatening as he began challenging himself with new motor plans: jumping and crashing into pillows, climbing up the vertical ladder or even crawling over the air mattress. Adam spoke, "Mama" and "Dada." His parents were overjoyed.

After about 12 weeks on a modulated music program, SAMONAS CDs were added. More intensive postural/respiratory activities were added to home activities.

After seven months, Jenny was excited as we spoke of all the changes Adam had made and what a journey it had been. "Adam has come so far, so fast," she began. No longer did he scream through the night. There was no more head banging or head hitting. Eye contact and interactive behaviors had significantly changed between mother and son. Jenny was visibly moved. Just recently Adam had begun to play with other children. He displayed an overall drive to explore his surroundings.

The acceleration in speech and language had been truly remarkable - Adam was now approximating 175 words. Previously feared tactile experiences such as sand-play or hair washing had become activities of delight. Cuts and bruises now had meaning to him - Jenny laughed as she described Adam's game as he'd fall and give a little cry asking his mother to kiss it better. "He's such a little actor now - he makes us all laugh" As we talked I watched Adam intermittently kissing and rubbing his mother's face with great joy and giggles. "It feels wonderful" said Jenny with a tear in her eye. And though there were bridges yet to cross, it was touching to see how far this little boy had come.

Bryce

Bryce was very much a loner and his parents were concerned about his lack of engagement. It seemed that his world and the world outside did not connect. Sometimes he would watch other children play but rarely did he choose to interact with them. He had a number of unusual sensory seeking behaviors, including opening and closing spring loaded doors creating a loud banging sound.

He began his Therapeutic Listening program with 4 weeks of modulated music and 4 weeks of SAMONAS. After that time, his mother spoke warmly as she described the changes Bryce had made. Actively initiating play with other children in the neighborhood was a positive change. She talked excitedly about how much more aware he was of people and the world in general. "We went outside and he immediately turned to the bird that was chirping. Another day he oriented to the fire engine outside. Bryce is orienting to sounds. This is new for us."

She talked about the tremendous increase in vocalizations, with babbling and baby talk. He began repeating words. Then it happened - spontaneously Bryce came to Suzanne saying "Mama." "I cried," she said. Bryce also began repeating his name.

Changes in perception were also noticed. Previously, when picture cards were displayed as a form of communication Bryce seemed unable to process their meaning. Then, Suzanne noticed, "When the picture was the cue to KICK, Bryce went over to the ball and kicked it. He never processed things like that before!"

Bryce's relationship to his body also began to change. A common pattern for him was standing on his toes in an extended posture with hands flapping beside him. Jumping was done with a retracted and extended body and all movements lacked control. "Suddenly I noticed him jumping in the pool," said Suzanne. "Something was different. Bryce was pulling up his legs and jumping in flexion!"

He started to use his upper body with more control. Previously, Bryce had made little use of his upper body. He never pushed up. He never crawled on all fours. He just stood upright and walked. "Whenever he fell he would not put out his hands to protect himself. This was one of the first things we noticed," Suzanne commented. Bryce had demonstrated no protective extension, but now Bryce began to notice the usefulness of his arms, hands and fingers.

Suzanne described changes in his fine motor skills as phenomenal. Scissors usage had always been a difficult for Bryce, requiring hand over hand assistance guiding his fingers through the process. "Now he is mechanically opening and shutting the scissors all on his own," his mother reports. Bryce had also been unable to hold a pencil with a functional grip, but recently, "He took the pen out of my hand and just automatically started drawing with the appropriate grip."

"I have seen dramatic changes in the way he carries himself" said Suzanne. Focus, attention span and following directions had been impressively impacted. His former ritalin dosage of 12 mg was dropped to 7 mg.

"The biggest change for him has been his awareness of other people and his understanding. Initially we thought that Bryce had auditory processing problems. We have since seen so much change, and not just the auditory processing. It's like the whole package has just changed. It's like having a whole different kid."

Johnny

My son Johnny is a bright, creative child. He was always good at playing independently. He was dressing by himself, building with Legos®, putting together train sets and writing his name when he was 2 years old. Socially, however, he appeared more withdrawn than other children his age, and often did not respond to others when they spoke to him. We began to wonder about his hearing, and when his preschool teacher mentioned concerns with his hearing as well, we decided to get a hearing evaluation by an audiologist. It turned out he had a moderate to severe hearing loss in both ears, due to fluid in his middle ear. Since he did not have speech delays, it was difficult to convince our pediatrician to refer us to an Ear, Nose & Throat (ENT) specialist. Once we did see an ENT, and after 6 months of allergy medication, Johnny had tubes placed in both ears. He then passed his hearing evaluation with normal hearing in both ears. He continued to excel in visual motor skills, however, his social skills appeared to be a struggle for him.

We then discovered he had highly superior intelligence following an evaluation by a school psychologist. She also noted that even though his scores were above average, he appeared to struggle with verbal tasks and excelled in visual tasks. She suggested we investigate educational programs designed for gifted children. Meanwhile, his new preschool teacher expressed concerns with Johnny's introverted social behavior, stating he was showing autistic-like behaviors. Since I am a pediatric Occupational Therapist, I knew my son was not autistic, and felt devastated that his behavior was so gravely misunderstood. Yet, we wondered why his social skills remained a struggle for him. I found myself constantly repeating what others would say to him several times before he would respond, if at all. He appeared so involved in what he was doing or thinking, that he seemed unaware of what was going on around him. At home, or in a quiet environment, he was so much fun to be around, and so creative. I wanted somehow to help him to share and interact that way in other environments. Things like birthday parties, park district classes and new situations appeared difficult for him. I also noticed that he never liked swinging, and was very cautious when moving around in his environment.

During his gym classes, he wandered around instead of following along with the other children. During soccer, he did the drills very well, however when it came to playing a game, he again would wander around the field instead of participating in the game. He now attends a private school for gifted education. At school, Johnny's teachers describe him as a bright and talented child, however, he can be "easily distracted or absorbed in his own thoughts and sometimes seems not to be paying attention." We also noticed that Johnny has difficulty shifting his focus, and communicating social/personal issues. When playing with friends, he has a hard time playing what they want to play. Instead he wants to play around themes of his strong interests. With a background in sensory integration myself, I often wondered how and if all these pieces fit together somehow with his sensory processing. When I discovered Therapeutic Listening, the pieces began to fit together.

After an evaluation with an occupational therapist trained in Sensory Integration and Therapeutic Listening, he began a listening program. He started with modulated music, which he accepted willingly and appeared to enjoy very much. He often would ask for the music, and request to do it while swinging or jumping on the trampoline. I began to notice immediate results. Just three days after he began on the home program, I observed him immediately respond to a neighbor who said hello to him. For the first time, I did not need to repeat or cue him to look up and say hello. He began noticing words that rhyme spontaneously during conversation, and began following directions after we stated them only once. He has been interested in playing board games, the correct way, instead of making up his own rules. It has been three weeks and we've seen amazing results from his listening home program.

On his follow-up visit at 4 weeks, he was much more engaged and interactive with the equipment and his therapist. He followed her directions the first time she stated them, without me repeating them. He appeared to pick up on social nonverbal interactions as well. Since then I've heard him say "I'm good at that" when he accomplishes something new. Johnny has never been a big risk taker, however, he recently began requesting to do more physical play (riding his bike, jumping on the trampoline, swinging). The highlight of our recent vacation, was Johnny rock climbing! It was amazing. He wanted to do it the minute he saw the wall, and after his third time, he wanted to go back the next day. The instructor was impressed that a five year old went half way up the wall, farther than his Mom and Dad! Not only did he climb well, but he interacted with his instructor (a stranger), and followed his verbal directions while climbing!

Adam's and Bryce's stories contributed by:
Genevieve Jereb, OTR, Madison, WI
Johnny's story contributed by his mother:
Susan Richey, MS, OTR/L

Listening with the Whole Body

The Purpose of this Book

The previous stories illustrate the power of incorporating sound based intervention strategies into occupational therapy treatment based on sensory integrative principles. This book is an attempt to share the information, experience and clinical reasoning that allowed the aforementioned children and many others to make dramatic improvements in life functions. The elements that support these changes are complex. We hope that this book will provide a structure for therapists to begin understanding and creating personalized programs for appropriate clients and their families.

As with any tool, application must be discrete and relevant to the individual. It is critical to understand the client's needs and to choose a listening protocol combined with overall treatment that matches those needs.

This work represents years of clinical practice with a variety of auditory interventions designed for numerous clients of all ages and abilities. Interaction with and mentoring of many therapists contributed to growth of knowledge and understanding of listening interventions. While there is a considerable amount of empirical research underway, current understanding is based on mounting clinical evidence reported in the United States and abroad.

The primary author, Sheila M. Frick has studied many sound therapy strategies and has developed a unique approach from her perspective as an occupational therapist with a sensory integrative frame of reference. The authors set forth guidelines (not rules) for use, to allow for the greatest possible clinical reasoning based on individual client needs and responses, as well as for growth and expansion of the work. They trust that every therapist will use this material responsibly.

Overview of Intervention with Sound

Hearing Versus Listening

Have you ever wondered how you know if someone is listening to what you are saying? It seems you can tell immediately if that person is truly "listening" to your words. Perhaps you have an intuitive sense about the complex process of "listening".........

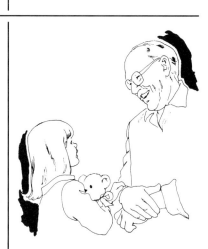

<u>Hearing</u> is passive. It is an involuntary act. Sound is received through the structures of the ear that pass it along like a microphone. The passive act of hearing does not involve the direction of attention to sound.

<u>Listening</u> is active. It is a voluntary act. Sound from the environment is selected for direct attention and focus. Active listening is dynamic and continually adapting. Listening requires the desire to communicate and the ability to focus the ear on certain sounds selected for discrimination and interpretation.

Perhaps you and parents and teachers have become adept at recognizing the difference between hearing and listening for a child. One would suspect that a child who is facing a parent or teacher, sitting upright, making eye contact, one ear slightly cocked in the direction of the adult's voice, body leaning toward the sound, is "listening." Why? One passively hears with the ear structures. One actively listens and directs attention to sound with the *whole body*.

Why is *listening* important? It is through listening that we are able to connect our inner and outer worlds. It is the most basic precursor to interaction, speaking, reading and writing. It relates closely to attention, focus, vigilance and concentration. Sounds provide information regarding time and space. Sounds provide us with an ability to categorize and organize perceptions. They magnify our window on the world.

An Historical Perspective of Listening Techniques

A growing number of occupational therapists and other professionals are incorporating sound based technologies and methodologies into their current practice. These sound-based stimulation programs combine the therapeutic benefits of music with sophisticated sound technology. Such tools enable therapists to approach the auditory system directly through the use of electronically altered music.

Sound therapy consists of equipment and materials that have been designed to produce specific effects on listening skills following a prescribed program. Listening difficulties (i.e. the ability to accurately perceive, process and respond to sounds) are often a part of other perceptual, motor, attention and learning difficulties that affect a large number of children and adults with sensory processing problems.

There are several sound based treatment methods available in the United States and abroad. The following is a short summary of various methods currently available and their historical relationship to each other.

TOMATIS

Tomatis originally defined the role of the ear as the "integrator," structuring organization at all levels of the nervous system (Thompson, 1991). He connected listening to the development of receptive and expressive language, learning, motor control and motivation. Tomatis developed Audio Psycho Phonology, listening training that is most commonly referred to as the Tomatis Method.

Dr. Alfred Tomatis, a French Ear, Nose and Throat specialist, was one of the first practitioners to develop an approach for treating listening difficulties. Tomatis originally defined the role of the ear as the "integrator," structuring neural organization at all levels of the nervous system (Thompson, 1991). He connected listening to the development of receptive and expressive language, learning, motor control and motivation. Through his clinical work with opera singers and factory workers, Tomatis recognized that the voice can only produce what the ear can hear, a principle now known as the 'Tomatis effect.' His study of the ear led to the conviction that, the overall function of the vestibulocochlear mechanism is to detect and analyze movement. He described the vestibular portion of the vestibulocochlear system as picking up and discriminating the larger movements of the body, which we can see and feel. Similarly, the auditory (cochlear) portion registers and differentiates the finer movements of sound waves, which pass through the air and are funneled into the ear (Madaule, 1993).

In the mid-1900s, Tomatis developed a listening technique to "reeducate the ear" based upon the following four principles:
_ Motivational and emotional needs begin with listening.
_ Listening plays a fundamental role in language.
_ The auditory system relates self to self, others and the universe.
_ The brain needs sound energy to enable the thinking process and the development of integration.
(as cited in Brewer/Campbell, 1991, p. 287)

Tomatis developed the first auditory training or listening training device, using progressively filtered sounds, specifically those sounds rich in high frequencies (i.e. classical music, the mother's voice, Gregorian chants), to effect change. Tomatis was the first to recognize the importance of high frequency audition. He spoke of high frequency sound as charging the brain. The Tomatis Method of auditory training is a clinic-based program, requiring the use of specialized equipment and the expertise of a practitioner trained in the Tomatis approach.

A listening program that may be used at home in some cases, Listening Fitness, is available in the United States and Canada. This program provides listening training using sound stimulation. It is designed by Paul Madaule who worked closely with Dr. Tomatis and has used the Tomatis Method for over 30 years. While Listening Fitness is based on some of the key concepts of the Tomatis Method, it differs substantially in assessment procedures, audio equipment and its targeted use. It can be a useful part of a treatment regimen where the goal is to help an individual to develop and improve both receptive and expressive listening. Like other listening techniques, Listening Fitness includes a passive phase of intervention. Unlike other auditory based home programs, Listening Fitness provides an active component or the 'expressive phase.' This is where one gains control over voice and body through voice exercises (humming, singing, reading into a microphone). The total program lasts about 10 weeks with usually one or two hours of listening a day and a short interruption between the two phases.

Paul Madaule has also developed a unique assessment tool, The Listening Identification System. It is designed to determine specific listening difficulties and provides valuable information for individualizing listening protocols (Madaule, 1999).

Listening Fitness Instructors are carefully screened and trained and are supervised for one year by a highly qualified training team of consultants from the Listening Centre in Toronto, Canada. Founded over 20 years ago by the Director, Paul Madaule, the author of *When Listening Comes Alive (Madaule, 1993)*, the Listening Centre is a leader in the field of listening therapy. Currently Listening Fitness is being used as an educational tool with children with listening and learning difficulties. Listening Fitness may also be part of a clinic based program.

Most of the clinically based auditory training techniques are based on the early work of Tomatis, including that of Dr. Guy Berard, a French physician who studied and worked with Tomatis. Berard felt that the original protocol of Tomatis was too lengthy and developed a different method of filtering sound. His technique, which uses filtered pop music in which sound frequencies are electronically distorted/modulated at random intervals for random periods of time, is called Auditory Integra-

MADAULE

Listening Fitness, designed by Paul Madaule, is based on 'key concepts' from Dr. Tomatis' work. It is directed toward the impact of listening on learning, academics and vocal expression. This program is also referred to as the 'LiFT.'

BERARD

Auditory Integration Training (AIT) was developed to improve auditory hyper-responsivity and/or distortions or delays in the signals that interfere with an individual's ability to process auditory information. The Berard Method uses electronically modulated pop music with narrow band filters to reduce distortions in 'hearing.'

tion Training (AIT). Berard believes that distortions in the 'hearing' causes auditory processing problems. Berard and his technique gained worldwide recognition in 1991 with the publication of Annabel Stehli's biographical account of her daughter Georgie. *The Sound of a Miracle* (1991) describes how Georgie, diagnosed with severe autism, greatly benefited from a course of 20 AIT treatments with Berard. AIT is a clinic based program; implementation relies upon the use of the Audiokinetron (a device developed by Berard for filtering music) and a practitioner with specialized training (Frick, Lawton-Shirley, 1994). Just recently, Berard has developed updated equipment, the Earducator. This updated version of AIT is available through trained practitioners.

Until recently, implementation of auditory techniques depended upon the use of specialized equipment that allowed the therapist to individually tailor the filtering process to an individual's hearing pattern. The expense of the equipment and training as well as the limits of intensive in-clinic treatment has proved prohibitive in accessing these techniques for many therapists and their clients.

With the advent of new technology, similar tools have become available on compact disc. Although *similar* they *do not* replace either the Tomatis Method or AIT. The compact discs do provide a less intense way to access the vestibulocochlear system to impact neural function and integration and are easily available to clinicians in a variety of practice arenas.

MUELLER

The modulation on the EASe discs is similar to AIT, but without the capacity to individually select a specific filter.

Bill Mueller, an American sound engineer, through his company Vision Audio, developed one such tool. Mueller serves on the Board of Directors for the Institute of Human Potential and created a CD that filters simple, electronic music through an auditory stimulation device onto compact discs. These discs utilize a form of modulation that he describes as transient auditory stimulation that creates a general modulatory affect. This modulation is similar to the modulation used in the Berard method (AIT) but without the capacity to individually select a specific filter. This disc program is called **EASe** and is suitable for home, school settings and clinical programs when prescribed and monitored by a knowledgeable clinician.

STEINBACH

Steinbach based his work on Tomatis' idea of the importance of high frequency audition. He emphasizes spatial components and the natural structure of music. His recordings may be used with various populations depending on the background and expertise of the practitioner. His method is known as SAMONAS Sound Therapy.

The **SAMONAS** method is another such tool, which has combined some of the ideas of Tomatis with advances in both technology and physics. This method was developed by Ingo Steinbach, a German acoustical physicist, who has a broad background in music, physics and electronics.

Steinbach pays close attention to the selection of the music and·instrumentation for therapeutic purposes. He feels strongly about using classical music for several reasons. He states, "music is like language, it expresses a certain message" (Steinbach, 2000). The classical composers had an in-depth knowledge of how to use the elements of melody, harmony and rhythm to express their ideas and feelings. Their music was used to express their ideas about the "creation of life and the beauty that exists in the world." Using Mozart as an example, Steinbach states, "Just by listening to Mozart's music we can experience elements of life which are far beyond words" (Steinbach, 2000).

Steinbach feels strongly that the music used in therapy needs to express a positive mood in order to engage the client and motivate him to "wish to make change." In addition, the elements in classical music are many and varied depending on the choice of music. "The variety of music used in SAMONAS becomes a toolbox from which each therapist must make his own choice." (Steinbach, 2000)

Along with classical music many of the recordings used in the SAMONAS system include nature sounds, broadening the choices and providing additional spatial elements that invite listening.

The production and recording processes are considered critical to the therapeutic value of the recording. Steinbach takes extreme care in every step of the recording process from the selection of the music to the selection of the instruments, musicians and location of the recordings. He uses only natural instruments that produce rich harmonic sounds, noting the difference in structure of the sound patterns between electronic and natural sounds. Electronic instruments produce sounds that have a relatively simple structure when compared to acoustical instruments. All of the recordings used for SAMONAS are recorded according to a special process that maintains the optimal natural structure of the sounds. This system makes it possible to preserve the valuable elements and structure of natural sounds and music throughout the entire process of recording, processing and reproduction.

Steinbach is convinced that we listen in three-dimensional space and therefore the space "must be preserved in the recording. The moment we start the recording process we take extreme care to include the vital element of space in all SAMONAS recordings." (Steinbach, 2000) He attends to the acoustical qualities of the space, its size and expansiveness. A critical element in this spatial recording process is the clear preservation of the reference point of the listener. This point " differentiates between the individual and the outside world."

Comparison of Listening Programs*

Listening Program	Tomatis	Listening Fitness	AIT	SAMONAS
Originator	Dr. Alfred Tomatis France	Paul Madaule Canada	Dr. Guy Berard France	Ingo Steinbach Germany
Formal Name of Technique	Tomatis Method Audio Psycho Phonology "Listening Training"	Listening Fitness (LiFT) "Listening Training"	Auditory Integration Training (AIT)	SAMONAS Sound Therapy
Theory	Developed theory regarding the development of hearing in utero and the impact of auditory stimulus on all aspects of development including movement processing. Recognizes sensory integrative value of auditory stimulus.	Based on 'key concepts' from Tomatis and directed toward the impact of listening on learning, academics and vocal expression.	Trained and worked with Tomatis. Developed his own device & protocol to reduce the time required to produce results. Emphasized auditory stimulus' impact on behavior and language.	Influenced by Tomatis and Temple Fay. Based on principles of music therapy in accordance with developmental aspects and natural laws of physics related to sound. Emphasizes the global impact of specific auditory stimulus on physical, emotional and energetic development.
Equipment	Electronic Ear; Headphones and bone conduction.	Portable audio processor (LiFT®), cassette player, tapes, headphone with microphone.	Berard: Audiokinetron (EERS). BGC: BGC Audio-tone Enhancer. Both use headphones of precise specifications and music approved for AIT.	CDs; headphones of precise specifications & bone conduction. Variety of other equipment for working with special populations.
Assessment	Listening test for auditory responses to a broad spectrum of frequencies through both air and bone conduction. Extensive evaluation of posture, psychosocial function, voice, learning, academics & laterality.	Developmental history. Listening Identification System developed by Paul Madaule. Relevant information (tests, school records) gathered by the practitioner.	Developmental History & current performance. Auditory threshold sensitivity (audiogram) and other auditory assessments performed by an audiologist.	Order threshold; dichotic listening test; SCAN and other assessments appropriate to the tester's profession.
Music	Audiotape recording of music by Mozart, Gregorian Chants, Mother's voice.	Mozart, Gregorian Chant, voice.	Approved music contains lively music with a broad range of frequencies processed through the AIT device.	Classical music and nature sounds.

Listening Program	Tomatis	Listening Fitness	AIT	SAMONAS
Modality	1. Gating mechanism modulates sound between high and low channels. 2. Hi-pass filters which eliminate all sounds below specific sound frequencies, e.g. when filtered at 2,000 Hz, the listener hears all frequencies above 2,000 Hz. 3. Balance control. 4. Bone and air conduction.	1. Gating mechanism modulates sound between high and low channels. 2. Hi-pass filters which eliminate all sounds below specific sound frequencies, e.g. when filtered at 2,000 Hz, the listener hears all frequencies above 2,000 Hz. 3. Balance control. 4. Air conduction.	Berard 1. Modulates (distorts) high/low frequencies quickly. 2. Can filter out specific sound frequencies. 3. Air conduction (headphones). BGC 1. Modulation is random. 2. Can filter out specific sound frequencies. 3. Air conduction (headphones).	1. Spatially enhanced recordings. 2. Spectrally activated music emphasizing harmonic structures (i.e. electronic envelope shape modulator that emphasizes the time differences in the shape of sound. 3. High extensions - short passages of high pass filtering which eliminate all sounds below specific frequencies. The degree of filtering progresses with higher levels of activation. 4. Air and bone conduction. 5. Possibility to request individualized CDs.
Program Duration	Two hours of listening per day is common in the first two phases. Between 30-40 hours with breaks for integration.	Non-intensive program: 30 hours over 10 weeks (1 hour/day for 6 out of 7 days). Intensive program: 60 hours with a break for integration.	Two half hours per day; total of 10 hours; completed within 12 days.	Daily use for an extended period of time. Variety of CDs available. Must be under supervision of a trained individual.
Where?	Applied in clinic.	Applied in clinic, school or at home.	Applied in clinic or school.	Applied at home and in clinic, or school.
Training Requirements	Extensive training provided by the Tomatis organization.	Experienced practitioners receive a three day training course - supervision & support with ten clients (12 to 18 months) for certification.	Professionals with experience or advanced degrees are trained by an approved professional trainer.	Entry level: Listening with the Whole Body course. Five day core training course; One year practical experience followed by written documentation and case studies.

* Adapted from work by Nancy Lawton-Shirley.

Steinbach discusses this spatial element in relationship to the development of time and space concepts as well as bilateral development. "We must be able to perceive from one point to be able to make sense out of right /left, front/back, top/bottom and far/near." He also points out that "space is the basis for the organization of time" (Steinbach, 2000). We link time together with the experience of space, i.e. it takes time to travel through space. We first need to experience space before we can establish time, planning and organization. Each recording then reflects the qualities of the space in which it was recorded, from the expansiveness found in many of the nature recordings, to the more well defined boundaries of castle walls which are reflected in the recording of a live performance of chamber music.

Steinbach also pays close attention to the emotional state of the musicians. Again, using the guiding principles of physics along with his musical background, he points out that sound is the 'carrier wave of intention.' He will only record the musicians when they are playing from a sense of joy. Although the technical skills of the musicians are apparent, Steinbach believes that the joyful nature of the musicians and their ability to play and relate to each other creates music that expresses intense joy.

Once the recording process is complete, Steinbach processes some of the recordings on special equipment that has been designed to intensify the high frequencies in the sound structure. Although this idea is based on some of the ideas of Alfred Tomatis, Steinbach's manner of activation is unique and provides a tool that can be utilized in combination with other sound technologies. A special device called the 'envelope shape modulator' enhances the upper frequency range, which activates the recordings. (Thus the acronym SAMONAS: Spectrally Activated Music of Optimal Natural Structure.)

Steinbach creates several different levels of recordings with varying intensities of spectral activation and filtering. The less intense compact discs are available to therapists with an understanding of the implication of filtered sound and its impact on the entire nervous system. The more intense compact discs require a longer more, intensive training period which provides the therapist with more advanced information regarding sound and training in the more sophisticated pieces of equipment used in SAMONAS Sound Therapy.

Therapeutic Listening™

Listening is a function of the entire brain and goes well beyond stimulating the auditory system. We listen with our whole body. In order to fully address listening difficulties one must also attend to the listening functions of both the hearing ear and the body ear. One such approach that addresses the multiple facets of listening is Therapeutic Listening.

Therapeutic Listening uses sound in combination with sensory integrative treatment techniques, emphasizing vestibular activities directed towards the integrating functions of the vestibular structures and the outcomes they support. Therapeutic Listening selectively combines a number of electronically altered compact discs, based on the ideas and the technology created by Alfred Tomatis, Guy Berard and Ingo Steinbach, within a Sensory Integration frame of reference. These discs vary in musical style, quality of sounds and level of enhancement. Individual listening programs are created to address each client's specific problem. The choice of music and type of modulation, as well as listening time and accompanying individualized activity program varies depending on the treatment goals of the client.

When a Therapeutic Listening program is being implemented, as with all interventions based on the principles of Sensory Integration, a therapist relies on the client's cues to determine appropriate strategies (Kimball, 1993). Activities that are centered on postural activation and organization and oral motor and respiratory strategies are often a part of each client's program. These are important components of adaptive responses, which support CNS organization furthering the refinement of listening functions.

A client (especially a child) may be very active while listening, working on suspended equipment and three dimensional surfaces, which further challenge postural organization, motor planning and higher-level sensory integration skills (Fig. 1-1). The use of sound and music is so intimately connected to movement that children on listening programs are often compelled to move and explore the environment in new ways. It is not uncommon to see immediate changes in components of movement such as righting reactions, equilibrium, emerging stability/mobility and bilateral movement patterns.

The sound stimulation used in Therapeutic Listening is designed to set up the nervous system and prepare it for emergent skill. Skill may appear in a variety of areas. It is critically important to provide opportunity for exploration and mastery of skills as they emerge. Providing the 'just right' challenge and plenty

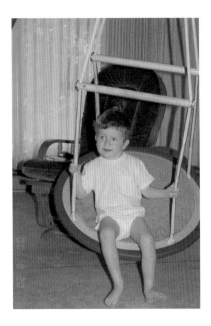

Fig. 1-1

of opportunities for repetition and variation allow the skills to become readily accessible. As mentioned earlier it is generally critical to provide specific postural, movement and respiratory activities as part of a program. Gaining postural organization (midline organization, dynamic co-contraction and bilateral integration) is often the "glue" that allows other changes in movement and sensory modulation for meeting and adapting to the opportunities and challenges of daily life.

Fig. 1-2

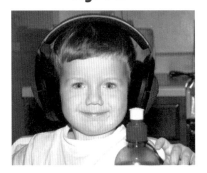

Since Therapeutic Listening does not involve sophisticated equipment, a prescribed program can be carried out at home, in school, or in the clinic (Figs. 1-1 & 1-2). Many school-based therapists have set up and monitored a program that is carried out in the classroom along with other therapeutic activities. A typical program may be in place for two to six months for initial gains; however many individuals continue past this time frame or find several compact discs useful as part of an ongoing "sensory diet" (Wilbarger & Wilbarger, 1991).

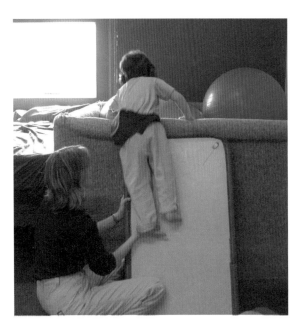

Fig. 1-3

Clients with a number of developmental and acquired difficulties have benefited from a Therapeutic Listening program. Sound appears to be a very powerful way to access both portions of the vestibulocochlear system. It is important to realize that this system works to process sensations of movement and sound (Fig. 1-3). The vestibular portion orients the body to place while the auditory portion localizes sounds and assists in navigating through space. Another related aspect of space, which is perceived by the system, is time. The vestibular portion perceives and coordinates the temporal (or timing) aspects of movement while the auditory portion perceives the temporal aspects of sound. The vestibular cochlear system plays a significant role in the perception of time and space that underlies the organization of sensory motor functions and form the basis for perceptual organization (Ayres, 1972; Madaule, 1993).

Although Ayres (1972) wrote about the relationship between the auditory and vestibular structures, she never directly addressed enhanced auditory input. Thus when Therapeutic Listening is done in the context of activities that require active involvement and adaptive interactions, it represents an expansion of interventions based on principles of Sensory Integration theory. However, when it is used alone, in the absence of any demand for adaptive interaction, it represents pure sensory stimulation and falls outside the context of Sensory Integration treatment principles. It appears that sound stimulation alone facilitates the process of listening and social engagement (Porges, 1997). However, to maintain and expand on those changes it is critical to engage the client in functionally and developmentally relevant activities that allow the changes to become a part of daily life skills.

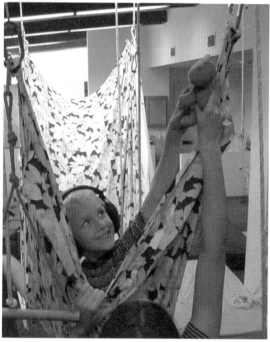

Fig. 1-4 (left)
While listening to a prescribed CD, this child is climbing in a lycra swing, challenging and facilitating midline organization and postural adjustments.

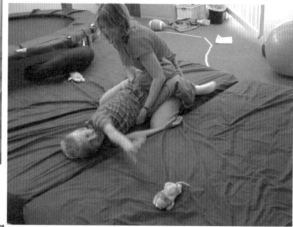

Fig. 1-5 (above)
Following the client's listening session, the occupational therapist uses 'hands on' play wrestling techniques to refine posture, combined with visually directed reach.

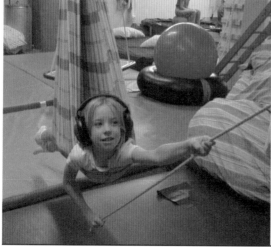

Fig. 1-6 (left)
This child engages in functional activities that allow her to make an adaptive response while listening to the prescribed CD.

Current clinical work suggests that Therapeutic Listening decreases the time necessary to meet treatment goals (Frick, Jetter, Volpe, and Redner, 2001). When incorporated into a Sensory Integrative treatment approach, changes are typically observed in:

- attention
- organization of behavior
- self regulation
- development, refinement and mastery of postural and motor skills
- bilateral motor patterns
- articulation
- emergence of praxis
- fine motor skill

(See Chapter 4: Clinical Reasoning and Documented Outcomes).

Other clinical outcomes that reflect improved spatial temporal organization are seen functionally in handwriting and visual motor skill; timing of motor execution; improved timing in social interactions; and discrimination of the dimensionality and directionality of spatial concepts. Since many of these skills support communication it is not unusual to see improvement in many components of communication, such as a greater range of nonverbal communication, greater emotional and verbal expression and improvements in pragmatic language. Many of the above mentioned clinical outcomes occur within a short period (hours, days, weeks) of initiating a Therapeutic Listening program.

The Relationship of Listening to Sensory Integration

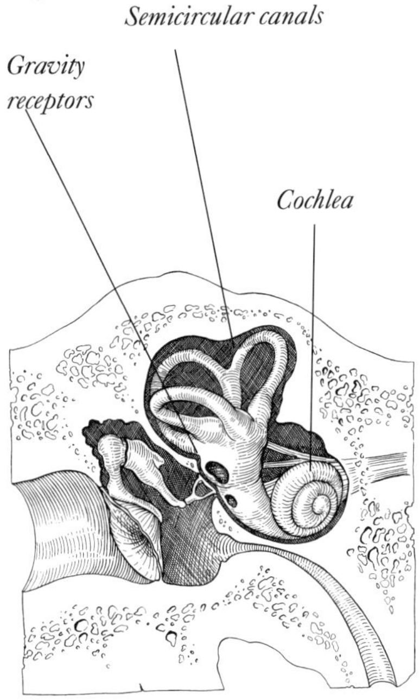

The outcomes observed with the addition of Therapeutic Listening are not surprising to those therapists who are familiar with the sensory integrative process and its resultant clinical outcomes.

All of the senses (touch, movement, smell, taste, hearing and vision) facilitate an individual's understanding of the world and enhance skill development. Dysfunction in the processing of sensation the senses can impact many areas of development and function. Sensory integration affects changes at the level of the brainstem (Ayres, 1972; Cool, 1987), as does Therapeutic Listening. Listening is related to arousal, self-regulation, emotion, respiration, postural adaptation, visual motor skills and oral motor skills through the interconnected neuroanatomy of both portions of the vestibulocochlear system (Fig. 1-7).

Ayres (1979) and other investigators of the vestibular portion of the system have shown that it is instrumental in supporting the functions of:

Fig. 1-7

Semicircular canals

Gravity receptors

Cochlea

- Orientation to gravity.
- Awareness of movement through space.
- Influencing antigravity muscle tone.
- Coordinating head and eye movement.
- Coordinating the two sides of the body.
- Arousal, attention and self-regulation.
- Integrating all sensory systems for organization.
- Developing body scheme.

The auditory/vestibular system functions to provide perception of time and space, the reference point from which all sensation is organized (Ayres, 1972; Tomatis, 1991).

Ayres pointed out the primacy of auditory input in the orienting response. She classified the brain's processing of sound as "one of the primal forms of sensory integration." She describes the auditory portion as having "primal significance to survival" and thus having influence over "several integrating neurons at the brain stem and other subcortical locations" (Ayres, 1972, p. 71). From Ayres' perspective, both an individual's survival and discriminative functions could be impacted by treatment aimed at enhancement of vestibular-auditory processing.

The auditory/vestibular system is often viewed and discussed as two distinct systems. The cochlea, in terms of its ability to process sound, has been studied by neuroscientists. Meanwhile, the vestibular system has been studied by occupational therapists in relation to perception of movement and contributions to learning. Early on, Ayres (1979) looked at the functional relationships between the vestibular and cochlear portions. She described improvements in auditory processing skill in the children she was treating with sensory integrative techniques that incorporated strong vestibular input. She discussed both the vestibular and auditory portions as having a powerful impact on efficient neural processing. In doing so, she noted the important integration of information from the vestibular portion in subcortical processing centers that is necessary for auditory input to have meaning. Based on this observation she recommended incorporating strong vestibular input into treatment strategies to enhance auditory processing and language related learning difficulties.

Comment from Dr. Ayres at a panel discussion on control of sensory input: "... I have always been a little reluctant to use passive stimuli, but now I am fairly convinced that bombardment of vestibular stimulation may make the nervous system more receptive to auditory stimulation and able to do a better job of processing it. Therefore, I use passive stimuli in order to get the nervous system into a state that the child can't bring about by himself."
(In Henderson & Coryell, 1973. p. 139)

The relationship of auditory processes and functioning to sensory integration lies in the anatomy and phylogeny of the vestibulocochlear structures. They both share the bony labyrinth of the inner ear. Their mechanical receptors operate in very similar fashion, with common fluids - the perilymph and endolymph and they share a common cranial nerve (VIII), of which, even some of the fibers appear to be shared (Moore, 1973).

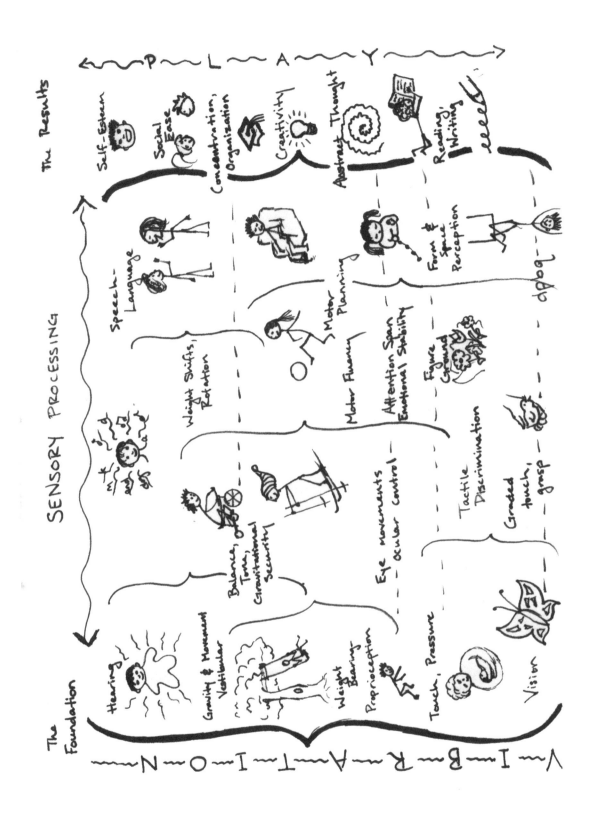

A pictorial representation of the impact of vibration from music and sound on the sensory integration process. By Lois Hickman, 1997, from the course: Accelerating sensory integration through stories, games and musical play. Austin, TX. Printed with permission.

Listening with the Whole Body

Moore (1979) discussed the close functional relationship between these structures. She stated that phylogenetic studies demonstrate that the two systems developed as a unit and appear to be connected from both a structural and functional point of view. She pointed out the close relationship between the gravity receptors and the cochlea.

The auditory structures are an evolutionary partner of the vestibular structures which evolved to pick up the finer movements of the oscillating air molecules that create sound. Because of this partnership, we must also consider this portion of the vestibular cochlear system's influence on refining and elaborating the above mentioned functions of the vestibular system along with its obvious ties to language and communication functions.

Interestingly, the earliest auditory structures evolved in primitive fish as a group of hair cells emerging out of the top of the gravity receptors. It is believed this evolution was a response to the need to communicate with other fish. Such communication required the ability to pick up finer vibrations in the water. The auditory structures became more sophisticated as the species moved up on land, initially using the bones in the jaw to transmit the low frequency vibrations from the ground to the inner ear. This portion of the system needed further refinement, developing the structures of the middle ear out of the now unneeded length of jaw bones, as mammals evolved to progressively assume more of a vertical orientation. They then required the detection of finer and finer vibrations of vocal communication and eventually spoken language which are transmitted through the air.

In other words, there is a close relationship between the receptors that are responsible for orienting our body in space (vestibular) with the receptors that orient us to the environment (cochlear). These two senses are intimately tied to each other for accurate perception of the environment. Without accurate orientation of our bodies in space, we are unable to make sense out of sounds coming from the environment.

Tomatis (as cited in Madaule 1993, 1999) noticed the clinical connection between these two systems when he observed changes in vestibular related function (posture, movement and visual skills) while using sound stimulation in the treatment of a number of individuals with listening difficulties. He not only acknowledged the strong connection between these structures, but he viewed them as having the same function: the perception of movement. Madaule described the vestibular system as the "ear of the body" (p. 51) perceiving the slower movements and position of the body (low-frequency vibrations), whereas the cochlea perceives the faster oscillatory movements of airborne higher frequency vibrations.

When one looks at movement and sound as vibration and considers them from the point of view of physics, there appears to be no distinct point at which movement becomes sound. The only difference between movement and sound is the velocity of the vibrations. The transition from movement to rhythm to a tone is seamless (Steinbach 1997). This seamless transition is mirrored in the receptors of the vestibular and auditory structures. The slower vibrations that we can both feel and hear are received by both the vestibular and auditory systems.

Sound appears to be a very powerful way to stimulate both the vestibular and auditory structures. It is important to remember that both structures work together to process the sensations of movement and sound. The vestibular portion receives messages from the body about its position in space at any given moment and in any given position. The auditory portion receives and processes the finer movements of air molecules, sound, which we cannot see or feel but which orient us to and help us locate objects and sound producing events in the environment. Without accurate orientation of our bodies in space, we are unable to make sense out of the sounds coming from the environment. The vestibular portion of the vestibulocochlear system orients the body in space while the auditory portion helps us to orient to the surrounding space and navigate through it.

It is important to note that when the vestibulocochlear system is addressed in accordance with its relationship to functional skill in treatment, the impact appears to be greater than when these two modalities are addressed as separate, unrelated systems.

Another related aspect of spatial perception, provided by this system, is time. The vestibular portion perceives and coordinates the temporal (or timing) aspects of movement while the auditory portion perceives the temporal aspects of sound. The system plays a significant role in the perception of time and space that underlies the organization of sensory motor functions and form the basis for perceptual organization.

The vestibulocochlear system sets up the individual for focused attention in the environment and meaningful behavior and interaction with the environment. It is important to note that when the vestibulocochlear system is addressed in accordance with its relationship to functional skill in treatment, the impact appears to be greater than when these two modalities are addressed as separate, unrelated systems.

Many therapists currently trained in Therapeutic Listening find it an important addition to their Sensory Integration treatment modalities that can increase the intensity and shorten the duration of treatment.

References/Suggested Readings

Ayres, A. J. (1972). *Sensory integration and learning disorders.* Los Angeles: Western Psychological Services.

Ayres, A. J. (1973). In A. Henderson, & J. Coryell, (Eds.) *The body senses and perceptual deficit.* Boston: Boston University.

Ayres, A. J. (1979). *Sensory integration and the child.* Los Angeles: Western Psychological Services.

Berard, G. (1993). *Hearing equals behavior.* New Canaan, CT: Keats.

Brewer, C. & Campbell, D. G. (1991). *Rhythms of learning.* Tucson, AZ: Zephyr Press, Inc.

Cool, S. J. (1987, June). A view from the "outside": Sensory integration and developmental neurobiology. *Sensory integration Special Interest Section Newsletter,* 2-3. Rockville, MD: American Occupational Therapy Association.

Frick, S. M. & Lawton-Shirley, N. (1994, December). Auditory integrative training from a sensory integrative perspective. *Sensory Integration Special Interest Section Newsletter, 71* (4), 1-8.

Frick, S. M. (1999). SAMONAS sound therapy. *The Sound Connection,* 7(1), 1-2.

Frick, S. M. (2000, Spring/Summer). An overview of auditory interventions. *Sensory Integration Quarterly.* 1-3. Torrance, CA: Sensory Integration International.

Frick, S. M., Jetter, T., Volpe, P., Redner, L. (2001). Case studies in therapeutic listening *Therapeutic Resources Newsletter, Vol. I.* Madison: Therapeutic Resources.

Frick, S. M. (In Press). Therapeutic Listening. In A. G. Fisher, E. A. Murray & A. C. Bundy. *Sensory integration theory and practice, 2nd Ed.* Philadelphia: F. A. Davis.

Kimball, J. G. (1993). Sensory integrative frame of reference. In Kramer, P. & Hinojosa, J. (Eds.) *Frames of reference for pediatric occupational therapy.* Baltimore, MD: Williams & Wilkins.

Klangstudio LAMBDOMA (2000, August 11-17). *SAMONAS sound therapy theoretical concept and practical application.* Course manual. Madison, WI.

Madaule, P. (1993). *When listening comes alive: A guide to effective learning and communication.* Norval, Ontario: Moulin.

Madaule, P. (1997). *Listening training for children: Method, application and outcomes.* Paper presented at the meeting of The Interdisciplinary Council on Developmental and Learning Disabilities, Washington, D.C.

Madaule, P. (1999). *The listening fitness™ instructor's manual.* Toronto, Canada: The Listening Center.

Porges, S. (1997). *The listening project.* Paper presented at the meeting of The Interdisciplinary Council on Developmental and Learning Disabilities, Washington, D.C.

Stehli, A. (1991). *The sound of a miracle.* New York: Avon.

Steinbach, I. (1998) 3rd Ed., revised. *SAMONAS sound therapy: The way to health through sound.* Kellinghusen, Germany: Techau Verlag. (Original work published in German, 1994)

Steinbach, I. (2000, August). *SAMONAS sound therapy, theoretical concept and practical application.* Presentation: Core Seminar, Madison, WI.

Tomatis, A. A. (1991). *The conscious ear.* Station Hill Press.

Thompson, B. M. (1991). Listening disabilities: The plight of many. In A. Wolvin & C. Coakley, (Eds.) *Perspectives in listening.* Phoenix, AZ: Ablex Publishers.

Wilbarger, P. & Wilbarger J. (1991). *Sensory defensiveness in children ages 2-12; An intervention guide for parents and other caretakers.* Santa Barbara, CA: Avanti Educational Programs.

Wilson, T. (1991). Chant: The healing power of voice and ear (An interview with Alfred Tomatis, M.D.). In D. Campbell (Ed.), *Music: Physician for times to come* (p. 11-28). Wheaton, IL: The Theosophical Publishing House.

Windeck, S. L. & Laurel, M. (1989, March). A theoretical framework combining speech-language therapy with sensory integration treatment. *Sensory Integration Special Interest Section Newsletter*, p. 1-5. Rockville: American Occupational Therapy Association.

Structural & Functional Aspects of the Vestibulocochlear System

2

By Sheila Frick and Mary Kawar

Structures of the Ear and Their Functions

The auditory portion of the vestibulocochlear system is comprised of three structural components, divided by the tympanic membrane (ear drum) and the oval window. The first component, the outer ear, is designed to capture and reverberate sound from the environment and funnel it into the ear drum. The middle ear is the second component where two muscles modulate sound as it travels along the three ossicles (bones) from the tympanic membrane to the oval window. The third component is the inner ear which contains cochlear and vestibular mechanoreceptors designed to register and transduce sound and movement signals into electrical impulses. These impulses are conducted through the vestibulocochlear nerve (Cranial Nerve VIII) into the brainstem and throughout the central nervous system (CNS) where they are translated and integrated into meaningful and purposeful behavior involving arousal and attention, survival skills, postural control, communication, movement through space, spatial localization, and emotional tone.

Sound frequencies are altered as they travel through each part of the auditory mechanism so as to improve fidelity, particularly in the range of high frequency tones. Clarity in the higher frequency sounds, especially in the speech range and above, provides fine, detailed discrimination of voice intonation contours so as to recognize the speaker and interpret the speaker's emotional content. Fidelity also affords efficient comprehension of rapidly transmitted phonemes, the smallest segments of language, necessary for learning all aspects of language (speaking, reading and writing). Finally, the higher spectrum sounds provide discrete information about the direction of sound and the space in which it was produced.

Outer Ear

The outer ear consists of the pinna, the ear canal and the tympanic membrane. Air pressure waves (sound) captured by the

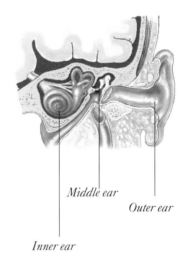

Middle ear

Outer ear

Inner ear

Fig. 2-1. Structures of the ear

pinna are amplified by its funnel-like design and the inch-long ear canal. Sound moves toward the tympanic membrane, causing it to vibrate upon contact. Pinna resonation enhances the high frequency sounds in the 4000 Hz range (upper range of a piano), a critical frequency for triggering attention (Steinbach, 1997; Madaule, 1993). The pinna, however, is too small to modify the long waves that are characteristic of sounds in the low frequency range (Schiffman, 1996). The length and shape of the ear canal creates resonance to enhance frequencies in the 3000 Hz range, key frequencies for recognizing voices. The tympanic membrane covers the entrance to the middle ear like the skin on a drum, with a similar vibratory capacity so as to project sound into the middle ear.

Middle Ear

The middle ear is an air-filled chamber that extends inward from the tympanic membrane to the oval window. The primary function of the middle ear is to transfer the vibratory movements of the eardrum to the fluid-filled inner ear. This is accomplished by mechanical conduction through three linked ossicles, the smallest bones in the body. They are the malleus (hammer), the incus (anvil) and the stapes (stirrup). Two striated muscles, the smallest in the body, are also located in the middle ear. The first of these muscles is the tensor tympani which is attached to the malleus to modify the tension of the tympanic membrane and thereby modulate incoming sound intensity as needed. The smaller of the two muscles is the stapedius which inserts into the stapes to accentuate high frequency sound as it is transmitted through the oval window into the inner ear. It is at the oval window that sound transmission must be converted from the ease of air conduction to the much greater resistance of fluid conduction. The mechanical linkage of the three ossicles is designed to generate the increase in energy (power) needed to conduct sound through fluid. This increased energy is transferred through the foot plate of the stirrup that is connected to the membrane of the oval window. This enhanced vibration then moves on into the perilymphatic fluid of the inner ear. It is noteworthy that, because of the orientation of the oval window, sound vibration is directed toward the saccule and utricle of the vestibular portion of the system *before* it moves on to stimulate the cochlea (Moore, 1972). This orientation of sound toward the vestibular receptors is perhaps a residual of an earlier stage of evolution when the saccule served as a primitive sound vibration receptor. It also suggests that the saccule and utricle may be vibratory receptors in addition to being movement and gravity receptors.

The two fold neuromuscular role of the middle ear muscles is to prevent sensory overload and to enhance sound discrimi-

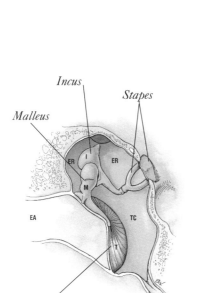

Incus

Stapes

Malleus

Tympanic membrane

Eustachian tube

Fig. 2-2. Middle ear ossicles

nation. Sound reduction is accomplished by reflex contraction of these muscles, about one tenth of a second after one or both ears are exposed to a loud, external sound. Just as the tiny pupillary muscles contract to control the amount of light that is permitted into the eyeball, the middle ear muscles contract to protect the delicate inner ear from excessive levels of sound. However, they cannot act fast enough to protect us from abrupt, transient sounds such as a gunshot. They are most effective in attenuating gradual onset, intense, low-frequency sounds, particularly those below 1000 Hz that are characteristic of naturally occurring sounds such as thunder. These muscles also protect the inner ear from fatigue and prevent sensory overload in the nervous system. Last but not least they contract to protect the individual from self-generated internal sounds. For example, they contract just before a person vocalizes to protect the system from the intensity of one's own voice. Without attenuation of the human voice, the shouting of a child would reach his or her ears at the same intensity as a train passing by (Borg & Counter, 1989). The internal noise of our own bodily functions needs to be screened as well. Individuals with paralysis, Bell's palsy (facial paralysis), for example, are often disturbed by popping or cracking noises as well as their own voice.

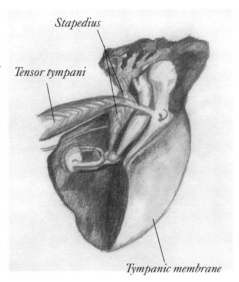

Fig. 2-3. Middle ear-tympanic membrane of ear drum

In addition to dampening loud internal and external sounds to prevent sensory overload, the middle ear muscles enhance sound discrimination. The stapedius, in particular is involved with increasing the fidelity of high frequency sounds. When the stapedius contracts, it mutes lower tones that tend to overpower the higher frequencies. In a sense, it acts as a dynamic filter that extracts speech from a noisy background. Counter & Borg's research (1989) has demonstrated that stapedius contraction enhances perception of the upper frequencies of sound, especially those in the speaking range, so that they are perceived as 50 dB louder.

The middle ear filter system is closely tied to our survival needs through core brain circuits that regulate emotion, arousal and attention. We easily tune in with our ears when something is meaningful, interesting or important to us. The muscles of the middle ear are influenced by descending projections from the cortex through attention and emotion centers. These connections can both increase or decrease contraction of the ear muscles as well as increase or decrease the sensitivity of the receptor cells of the cochlea. Netter (1986, p.178) points out that this is part of the brain circuitry in selective attention since "changes in the activity of the ear muscles have been observed during attentive behavior." When we are interested in something, these muscles work hard to filter out background noise so that we can easily tune in and listen to a sound source of interest. For example, the teenager readily tunes his ear to the discussion that he initiated about using the car. Conversely, the request to take out the garbage falls on deaf ears.

The muscles of the middle ear are also intimately connected with the parts of the nervous system that control facial expression, speech and visceral responses. There are several direct neurological interactions with functional ramifications between the ear and the four cranial nerves that supply the head and trunk, namely the trigeminal (V), facial (VII), glossopharyngeal (IX) and vagus (X) cranial nerves.

One very important interaction involves the trigeminal nerve (CN V) that is responsible for motor control of the jaw and sensation from the entire face well as motor control over the tensor tympani muscle of the middle ear. Since the tensor tympani is responsible for attenuation of sound, it is not surprising that auditorily defensive children have an intense need to chew, tense their jaw and/or grind their teeth when exposed to loud or noxious sounds.

Another interaction with clinical significance relates to the facial nerve (CN VII) that innervates the stapedius muscle of the middle ear as well as the muscles of facial expression. Closely tied to this, through neuroanatomical structures in the brain stem, is the glossopharyngeal nerve (CN IX) because of its control over the motor components of voice. Muscles designed to extract the human voice from a noisy background are thus linked with the muscles of facial expression and voice production that have such a powerful effect on non-verbal and verbal communication. During communication, we rely heavily on the non-verbal feedback that we pick up through the listener's facial expression. These same muscles are necessary for producing clear articulation and for hearing accurately and efficiently. Research has documented that children with poor auditory processing take up to 500 milliseconds to decipher a phoneme that should be processed in 40 milliseconds (Tallal, Miller, & Fitch, 1993).

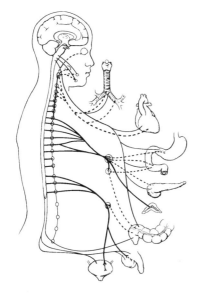

Fig. 2-4. Vagus nerve

Finally, the vagus nerve (CN X), that regulates automatic functions of the body (cardiac, respiratory, digestive and eliminatory), has a sensory branch on the tympanic membrane. This connection of the eardrum with visceral control of the pharynx and larynx influences our ability to speak and sing. The vagus nerve continues on to innervate the heart and lungs for physiologic regulation of arousal and attention and finally innervates the organs of the gut. The parasympathetic aspect of the autonomic nervous system has a key role in homeostasis, literally overseeing our gut reactions. The vagal system supports digestion, respiration and the regulation of emotional, motor and

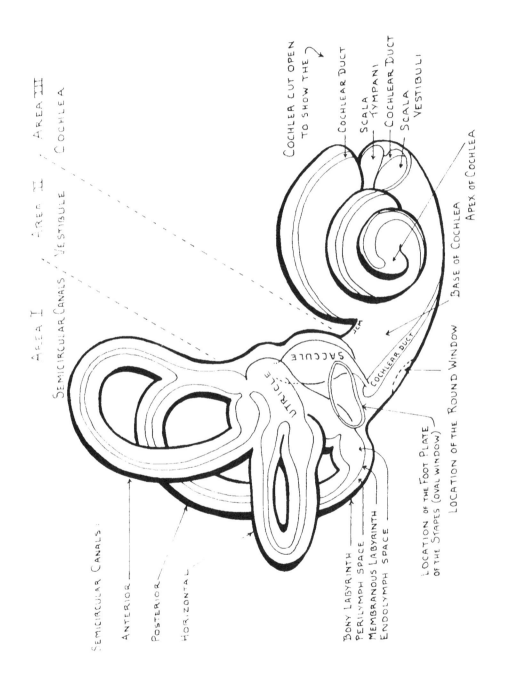

Fig. 2-5. From *The Body Senses and Perceptual Deficits*, Moore, J. 1972

J.C. Moore, Printed with permission.

vocal responses through its connections with the heart, lungs and oral structures (Porges, Doussard-Roosevelt, Portales, & Greenspan, 1996). The linkage of the ear with vagal nerve functions of self-regulation has profound therapeutic implications (see Chapter 3).

The middle ear is also connected by the eustachian tube to the pharynx. This connection helps to maintain appropriate air pressure in the middle ear. It can be a source of vestibulocochlear problems (i.e. ear infections, language and motor delays or disorders) that occur in infants and young children during critical developmental periods. Many of these children eventually present with sensory integrative dysfunction and learning disabilities. The eustachian tube lies in a horizontal position in infants and young children rather than at an angle that can provide good drainage as it does in the mature individual. (Oetter, Richter, & Frick, 1995). The horizontal orientation of the tube allows liquids to travel from the oral cavity into the middle ear where infection can subsequently develop. Infection often leaves sticky residue that decreases the efficiency of the middle ear muscles and bones to perform their designated functions. Children with vestibular hyporesponsivity, auditory processing problems, regulatory problems, articulation issues and/or oculomotor control problems are some of the diagnoses linked with a history of recurrent ear infections during infancy and early childhood. Other middle and inner ear problems can be precipitated by high fevers, allergies, trauma, restricted movement during in-utero development and chronic stress of the mother during pregnancy.

Inner Ear

Most neurology textbooks subdivide the inner ear into the vestibular structures and the cochlea, thereby treating them as two separate and distinct systems. There is a scarcity of resources that address the inner ear as a cohesive vestibulocochlear system with dynamic structural and functional interaction, essential for survival and sophisticated human performance. Together, these structures provide two ways of knowing about sound, movement and orientation in space. In essence, movement of the head stimulates the cochlea as well as the vestibular structures and sound waves stimulate the vestibular structures as well as the cochlea. The vestibulocochlear mechanisms are bilaterally represented in contralateral mirror image of each other, affording profound functional benefits through the system's ability to interpret the subtle but important differences between vestibulocochlear reception on one side compared to the other side.

It appears that nature has wisely protected the delicate membranous vestibulocochlear system by embedding it in the

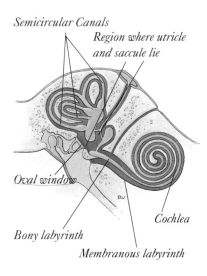

Semicircular Canals

Region where utricle and saccule lie

Oval window

Cochlea

Bony labyrinth

Membranous labyrinth

The continuous dark shading represents the space between the bony labyrinth and membranous labyrinth filled with perilymph.

Fig. 2-6. Inner ear

dense temporal bone. The space between the bony labyrinth and the membranous labyrinth is filled with perilymph. Endolymph flows within and throughout the membranous vestibulocochlear system. These watery fluids are the medium through which sound vibration, movement and gravitational influences are conducted so as to be registered by the mechanoreceptors. Bone conduction is another important medium for transmitting sound vibration into the fluid filled inner ear. Since bone conduction bypasses the middle ear, there are therapeutic implications regarding the use of bone conducted versus air conducted stimulation of the system.

The mechanoreceptors of the vestibulocochlear system deserve special mention as they are unique among all of the sensory receptors in the body. While most receptors in the body are designed to be more or less excitatory, each of the vestibulocochlear hair cell receptors has the capacity to decrease action potential firing rate when stimulated in one direction and to increase action potential firing rate when stimulated in the opposite direction. This duality of reception applies throughout the vestibulocochlear system in spite of the fact that there are a variety of hair cell designs within the system. Movement of the head to the left will increase action potential firing in cells of the vestibular organ on the right and decrease firing in the mirror image contralateral vestibular cells. Simultaneous, opposing signals from the two sides of the head is the fundamental, bilateral information needed for comprehension of movement stimulation. Similarly, sound stimulation of the cochlear hair cells in one direction increases cell firing and in the opposite direction decreases cell firing, depending on which direction the pressure from the endolymph flow causes the basilar membrane to bend.

Duality of vestibulocochlear sensory receptivity is made possible because of the arrangement of the fibers within the hair bundle that extend out of the top of each hair cell. Each hair bundle contains several stereocilia of varying length. These stereocilia taper toward a single, longer kinocilium. Bending of the stereocilia toward the kinocelium causes hyperpolarization (increased firing rate) of the cell body whereas bending of the stereocilia away from the kinocelium causes depolarization (decreased firing rater).

Fig. 2-7. Cochlea - uncoiled. From *The Body Senses and Perceptual Deficits*, Moore, J. In Henderson, Coryell, 1972.

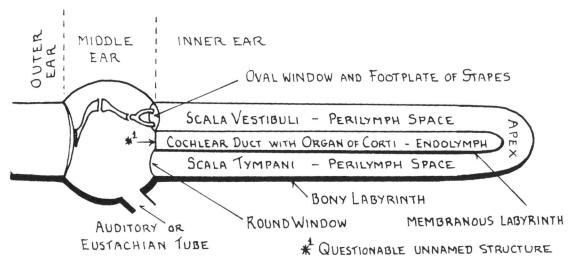

J.C. Moore, Printed with permission.

Vestibular Structures of the Inner Ear

The receptor end organs of the vestibular structures are contained within the bony labyrinth of the temporal bone, sharing the membranous labyrinth with the cochlea. Our dynamic, perpetual orientation in gravitational space is orchestrated through five different vestibular receptors. Two of these receptor sites are the otolith structures called the utricle and saccule which detect information regarding gravity and motion. They are capable of detecting linear acceleration along any axis. The other three receptor sites are the horizontal, the anterior vertical and posterior vertical semicircular canals. They detect rotary motion and angular acceleration around any axis. However, all five vestibular receptors work together in conjunction with the five contralateral vestibular receptors to keep us continuously informed about which way is up in the field of gravity, how our head is positioned at any point in time in three-dimensional space, what is moving, where we are going or being moved and how fast we are moving.

The utricle and saccule are fluid filled, oval sacs within the membranous labyrinth which contain thousands of hair cells, embedded in the base (macula) of each sac. At the top of each hair cell is a hair bundle that projects through the endolymphatic space into a gelatinous otolithic membrane on which calcium carbonate crystals called otoconia are embedded. Operationally, gravitational influences, head movement, bone vibration and/or low frequency sound result in slight displacement of the otolithic membrane, especially the loosely attached otoconia, causing the hair cell bundles to bend. As mentioned above, the direction of this mechanical bending determines whether the hair cell receives a signal to be mechanoelectrically transduced by the hair cells so that the vestibular nerve fibers can conduct this precise information on into the central nervous system.

As typical development proceeds the body becomes more and more adept at both moving and maintaining stillness relative to gravity. Without this gravitational reference point, orientation in auditory and visual space becomes disordered.

The utricle is oriented so that it primarily detects the magnitude and orientation of any acceleration in the horizontal plane. The saccule is oriented to detect vertical linear acceleration. As such, it is a primary gravity receptor site. Because gravity is a constant force its detection through the utricle and saccule provides necessary information for the development of antigravity postural control. This is accomplished by changes in the plane and direction of head movement during sensorimotor exploration and play. As typical development proceeds, the body becomes more and more adept at both moving and maintaining relative stillness because it is more accurately perceiving its motion and position relative to gravity. Without this gravitational reference point, orientation in auditory and visual space becomes disordered.

The horizontal, anterior and posterior semicircular canals are three fluid-filled tubes at right angles to each other, adjacent to the utricle. Interestingly, they are not positioned in the head's major anatomical planes of movement, but rather are offset so as to increase mechanoreceptor sensitivity to movement in "the x, y, z coordinate system of three dimensional space" (Cool, 1987). At the base of each canal is a thickened area called the ampullary crista that contains the hair cells. The hair bundles from each hair cell project into a gelatinous cupula that closes off a portion of the semicircular canal. Head movement displaces the canal endolymph in the opposite direction of the head turn once the fluid overcomes inertia. This displacement of fluid causes the cupula to be deflected, thereby bending the hair cell bundles in a positive or negative direction. This mechanical signal is transduced within the cell body, similar to the conversion of a mechanical signal into an electric signal by the utricle and saccule. When the head stops moving, the endolymph continues to move in the same direction. Steven J. Cool, PhD (2001), describes this phenomena as being similar to the movement of liquid in a cup on the console of a car wherein the liquid spills out over the back of the cup with forward acceleration of the car and over the front of the cup when the car stops. The semicircular canals primarily respond to changes in velocity along a curve so signals last only for the duration of the stimulation. The direction of head movement determines which of the semicircular canal signals is activated. This integrates the stimulation differences between the two canals for functional purposes such as ensuring that the two eyes maintain fixation on a visual target or sound source when the head turns.

Cochlear Structures of the Inner Ear

The cochlear portion of the inner ear is a one and one-half inch long tube that coils back on itself for two and one-half turns to form a snail-like structure. A cross-section of this tube reveals 3 chambers or canals that run the length of the tube. They are the upper vestibular canal which starts near the oval window and connects at the apex with the lower tympanic canal that ends at the round window. These two connected canals allow regulation of perilymph fluid displacement between the oval and round windows. The third canal is the cochlear duct that is sandwiched between the other two canals. It contains a specialized receptor structure consisting of the tough, yet flexible basilar membrane, the organ of corti, which rests on the basilar membrane and contains specialized sensory hair cells, nerves and supporting tissues for transforming mechanical impulses into electrical signals. Hair bundles extend out of the hair cells covering the basilar membrane. These hair bundles project through the endolymph filled space into the stiff tectorial membrane that protrudes above the organ of corti.

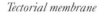

Tectorial membrane

Hair cells

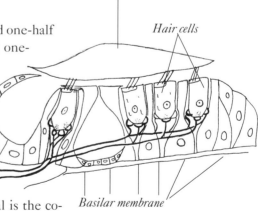

Basilar membrane

Fig. 2-8. Organ of corti

Movement of the stapes against the oval window results in vibration within the fluid filled cochlea, causing pressure differences between the scala vestibuli and tympani canals (see Fig. 2-7) that produce wavelike movement of the basilar membrane within the cochlear duct. Basilar membrane movement causes the hair cell bundles to bend against their attachment in the tectorial membrane. This bending is caused by a mechanical shearing force between the tectorial membrane and the basilar membrane. It is here that the signal is converted into an electrical potential to be carried through the cochlear branch of the eighth cranial nerve to the auditory nuclei in the brain stem.

The basilar membrane can be likened to a hairy xylophone with the hair cells being tonotopically arranged (cells that respond to similar sounds are placed next to each other). Sound frequency dictates the point that is stimulated along the basilar membrane. Each portion is set to respond to a specific frequency wave length. The longest, low frequency waves travel all the way to the apex of the cochlea, displacing the basilar membrane at its thickest, widest point. The short, high frequency waves vibrate the basilar membrane at the base of the cochlea, near the oval window, where the basilar membrane is thinnest and narrowest. Mid-range frequencies stimulate the mid-position of the basilar membrane. Tonotopic organization of sound frequency placement, starting at the nerve fibers along the basilar membrane, carries out all the way to the cortex to ensure organized, reliable discrimination and interpretation of sound frequencies. Approximately two-thirds of the hair cells are near the base of cochlea, providing more receptors to capture discrete differences in tones, especially the finer vibrations of higher frequency sounds. This leads to identification and detailed analysis of the sound source and the surrounding auditory environment. The higher frequencies of the sound spectrum have the capacity to energize us, elicit our attention and cue us to the details of the surrounding environment within which we are functioning at any given point in time.

Eighth Cranial Nerve (CN VIII)

The eighth cranial nerve contains a cochlear branch that connects the cochlear receptor end organs to the central nervous system and a vestibular branch that connects the vestibular receptor end organs to the central nervous system. These two branches have interconnecting fibers, underscoring the intimacy of the vestibulocochlear system regarding human performance and behavior. Within the vestibular branch there are separate subbranches for each of the semicircular canals and for the saccule and utricle. It is important to appreciate that, in addition to afferent fibers into the central nervous system, there are efferent fibers traveling from the central nervous system, including input from the contralateral cochlea and vestibular mechanisms, into the cochlea and vestibular mechanism which can modify the receptivity of the these end organs.

Phylogenetic-Ontogenetic Development

Phylogenetic studies suggest that the inner ear systems for hearing and orientation evolved from primitive sensory organs, capable of registering movement and vibration. The earliest fish had a group of hair-like receptors along the sides of their bodies that responded to the ripple in the water. These hair cells evolved over time to become fluid-filled membranes that migrated to the head of the fish (Ayres, 1979). The semicircular canals developed to provide directional information. As the fish became more sophisticated and the need arose to communicate with others, further adaptations were necessary to respond to the finer vibrations traveling through the water. In response to this need, additional groups of hair cells emerged from out of the top of the fluid filled sacs, becoming the early precursor of the gravity receptors. These hair cells were the first receptors for discriminating sound (Jourdain, 1997).

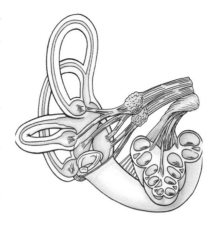

Fig 2-9. Vestibulocochlear divisions of the 8th CN

Further evolution facilitated the ability to survive on land. This new environment established a need for refinement of the structures to accommodate air conducted vibration of sound as well as fluid conduction.

The saccule served as a primitive hearing organ prior to the cochlea evolving as a more sophisticated mechanoreceptive system for capturing a wider range and more specificity of sound. Sound waves coming into the inner ear through the oval window are projected directly toward the saccule rather than toward the cochlea, implying an influence of sound on the vestibular system (Moore, 1972). The vestibular system responds to low frequency sound, thereby functioning as the 'ear of the body' (Madaule, 1993), while the high frequency sounds are the specialty of the mechanoreceptors of the cochlea.

Ontogeny recapitulates phylogeny as evidenced in the developing fetus. At four weeks of fetal development the auditory system and semicircular canals of the vestibular system emerge from otocysts (fluid-filled sacs containing the gravity receptors). The vestibular and cochlear systems develop and function interdependently to provide orientation and sound responsivity (see chart page 2-12). The importance of the inner ear structures is underscored by the fact that they are fully developed and functional by the fifth month in utero, prior to all other sensory organs. This early maturation of the vestibulocochlear system enables it to develop interconnections with the entire nervous system as it is elaborated over time.

Ontogenetic Development of the
Vestibulocochlear System

(from Elliot, 1999)
4 weeks fetal development -
The otocysts form (precursors of the utricle and saccule)

Auditory

6 weeks gestation - the auditory portion of the vestibulocochlear nerve forms

11 weeks gestation - cochlea emerges out of the top of the otocysts

10-20 weeks gestation - all 16,000 hair cell emerge in a gradient from the base to the apex

16 weeks gestation - all the relays to the inferior colliculus begin to myelinate (the inferior colliculus integrates information from sound with information about body position from the vestibular system for the purpose of orienting to sound)
- not fully myelinated until two years of age (refinement of this information happens throughout the sensorimotor stage of development)

Vestibular

5-10 weeks gestation - the vestibular tube emerges out of the bottom of the otocysts

7.5 weeks gestation - individual hair cell receptors develop in the vestibular receptor sites

8 weeks gestation - connections develop between 8th cranial nerve cells and the vestibular hair cell receptors

20-24 weeks gestation - beginning of myelinization due to the influence of gravity occurs in conjunction with myelinization of the nerves of the neck - the Moro Reflex can be elicited

24 weeks gestation - the cerebellum myelinates and connects with the vestibular structures for further integration and adaptation of vestibular senses with other sensory information

Early developing responses to sound are expressed through body movement. The fetus best distinguishes the frequencies from 20-12,000 Hz. Many of these frequencies also stimulate cutaneous and vestibular receptors.

23 weeks gestation- The fetus responds to sound by blinking and body movements.
24 weeks gestation - The fetus moves in rhythm to mother's voice.
(requires vestibular and cerebellar development)
28-35 weeks gestation - The fetus moves different body parts in response to different phonemes of mother's speech, demonstrating the ability to differentiate among speech sounds.

Central Processing of the Vestibulocochlear System

Sound and movement do not become meaningful information neurologically or behaviorally until they are received by several interactive systems within the brain that give meaning to the vestibulocochlear signals. Cochlear impulses are relayed through the cochlear branch of the eighth cranial nerve to the cochlear nuclei of the brain stem. Tonotopic order is maintained here as well as throughout the central nervous system. Vestibular impulses are relayed simultaneously to the vestibulocerebellum and to the brain stem vestibular nuclei through the vestibular branch of the eighth nerve. The brain stem continues the process of sorting, filtering and modifying sound and movement stimuli and facilitates their integration with all other functional aspects of human performance.

Central Processing of Vestibular Stimuli

The vestibular portion of the system is comprised of the peripheral apparatus, the vestibulocochlear nerve, the vestibular nuclei, the cerebellum and both ascending and descending fiber tracts. The vestibular portion is a master integrator of movement/gravity generated neurosensory information. Movement is an essential component of every aspect of life and gravity is a constant force.

Where there is life, there is movement. Therefore, the vestibular system plays a critical role in sensorimotor integration, albeit a role that may not be fully understood or adequately appreciated and, all too often, overlooked when dysfunction occurs. When functioning optimally, it provides us with:

◆ a primal sense of security and feeling of connectedness with the earth's surface through the details of postural orientation relative to the gravitational field.

◆ gaze stabilization despite head movement.

◆ the rate, extent and type of movement through space and time.

◆ registration and interpretation of low frequency sound.

◆ regulation and integration of movement with all types of sensory information.

◆ influence on the level of arousal and attention.

The vestibular mechanism has well defined sensory end organs, already discussed. Nerve fibers from each of the five vestibular end organs converge to form the vestibular branch of the eighth cranial nerve that sends signals to the ipsilateral and contralateral vestibular nuclear complex in the dorsal pons and medulla of the brain stem. There is a simultaneous direct connection between the end organs and the cerebellar flocculonodular lobe (vestibulocerebellum). Once vestibular input reaches the brain stem nuclei, it becomes unique among all other sensation because it influences both sensory and motor tracts. The efferent descending tracts from the vestibular nuclei influence motor behavior and the ascending tracts are afferent sensory projections. For this reason, Dr. Ayres (1972) referred the vestibular system as a "sensory-motor bridge system." The vestibular nuclear complex receives somatic, reticular and cerebellar input as well as signals from the contralateral vestibular end organs. Therefore, vestibular signals exiting the vestibular nuclear complex to all levels of the central nervous system are no longer pure vestibular signals because of modulation and integration with these other systems (Cohen & Keshner, 1989).

The lateral nuclei send descending motor commands influencing postural patterns and reflexes of the body. Further information is sent from the lateral vestibular nuclei to the reticular formation, the cerebellum and the contralateral vestibular nuclei. It is believed that this nucleus integrates vestibular and central motor signals. Through the medial longitudinal fasciculus, signals are sent to the oculomotor centers for gaze stabilization and ocular motility during head and/or body movement. Signals are also sent to the spinal cord because of rotary acceleration influence on muscle tone and body alignment (see note at left).

Note:
Well-defined reflexes support vestibular interaction with the sensory motor system. Vestibulo-cervical and vestibulo-spinal reflexes impact motor control. The vestibulo-ocular reflex allow the eyes to maintain fixation on the target when the head turns or moves through space and the pre- and post-rotary nystagmus reflexes are elicited in an attempt to refocus on a stable point in space when there is prolonged rotation of the body. Signals from the three paired semicircular canals interact specifically with the six paired extraocular eye muscles through pathways which project from the vestibular nuclei into the three bilateral cranial nerve nuclei (III, IV and VI) that control the six extraocular eye muscles.

Turning the head to orient to a sound source, holding the eyes steady to watch a stationary or moving object and maintaining ocular fixation during head and/or body movement are three functions that depend on vestibulo-proprioceptive monitoring and control of dynamic head-neck-body alignment. The close vestibulocochlear interplay starts at the receptor level whereas the vestibulo-somatosensory and vestibulo-visual interplay is evoked within the brain stem. Movement of the head in any direction will cause functionally specific, reflexive and/or volitional, directional movement of the eyes. While there does not appear to be a specific vestibulo-auditory reflex, both auditory and vestibular inputs are very closely tied to the orienting reflex, mediated in the inferior colliculus, just as there are intimate vestibulo-visual ties in the superior colliculus. The vestibular nuclei have several different pathways that project to the thalamus. Most of the direction-specific thalamic neurons respond to proprioceptive as well as vestibular stimuli (Cohen & Keshner, 1989). From the thalamus, some of the fibers project to the cortex while others go to the caudate nucleus of the basal ganglia along with auditory projections to impact the kinetic motor control system.

As discussed above, there are many interactive vestibular, ocular, auditory, cervical and spinal reflexes that support subconscious adaptive postural performance in a dynamic environment. We are thus free to use our intellect for exploring, creating and executing complex, consciously driven endeavors. Motor experience validates and integrates sensations into meaningful perceptions, including body scheme awareness and a sense of centeredness in time and space. The vestibular system also has a cortical influence on limbic function that impacts our emotional tone, our drive and our sense of security.

To date, three small vestibulocortical projection areas have been identified in cats and monkeys but no primary vestibular cortical area has been identified. Only one of the three projections has been found in humans. This is a projection to the posterior parietal lobe (Cohen & Keshner, 1989) in a region devoted to the integration of auditory, visual and somatosensory maps. Cool (1987) describes a thoughtful view of vestibulocortical function as "the central integrator of all sensory and motor systems, providing the reference base against which all sensory input and motor output information *must* be evaluated. It is this fixed-point reference location that allows for efficient and effective interpretation of incoming information and planning of outgoing motor information." The vestibular system provides critical information about our specific location in the overall spatial map, where we are in relation to the sights and sounds of our world. Conscious awareness of oneself in time and space is a prerequisite for where we are going, moment by moment. Dr. Cool, in a 2001 lecture, graphically described the vestibular posterior parietal projection as "your very own mall marker on the mall map of your life." Without this personal "you are here" arrow, you are literally lost in space.

Other sensory systems can compensate for inadequate or disordered vestibular processing, but not as automatically or efficiently. Less than optimal vestibular processing is particularly devastating in an immature nervous system because it has not had the opportunity to integrate information from all the senses for solid conceptual development. Perhaps the most exciting finding to date is that there are many ways into the system through multiple interconnected neuroanatomical structures. For example, a trial of Therapeutic Listening has been found to enhance balance and other vestibular related functions, just as a program that includes specifically designed movement and gravity activities has been found to enhance auditory processing. Combining well designed, individualized programs exponentially affects therapeutic outcomes. These therapeutic breakthroughs inspire us as clinicians to continue to hone our observation skills, be responsibly adventuresome in our treatments and share our failures as well as our insights.

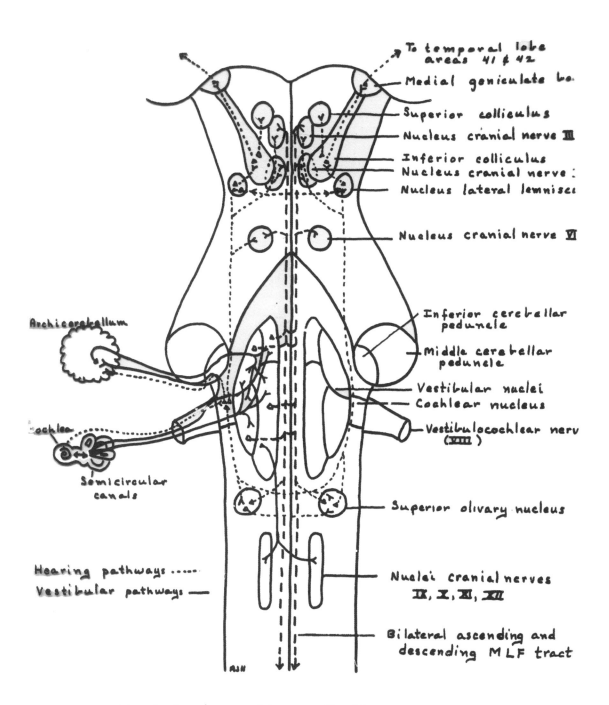

To temporal lobe
areas 41 & 42
Medial geniculate bo.
Superior colliculus
Nucleus cranial nerve III
Inferior colliculus
Nucleus cranial nerve :
Nucleus lateral lemnisci

Nucleus cranial nerve VI

Inferior cerebellar
peduncle
Middle cerebellar
peduncle
Vestibular nuclei
Cochlear nucleus
Vestibulocochlear nerv
(VIII)

Superior olivary nucleus

Nuclei cranial nerves
IX, X, XI, XII

Bilateral ascending and
descending MLF tract

Archicerebellum

Cochlea

Semicircular
canals

Hearing pathways ......
Vestibular pathways ——

Vestibulocochlear Pathways

Fig. 2-10.

J.C. Moore, Printed with permission.

Central Processing of Sound

A large amount of auditory information is processed at the level of the brain stem and other subcortical structures before it is passed on to the cortex for further refinement, discrimination and synthesis. Brain stem processing can be organized into two functional systems. One is the afferent auditory pathway that is comprised of thoroughly researched nuclei, relay stations and tracts that are concerned with what a sound is and from what direction is it coming. The other is the diffuse auditory system that is concerned with sound from an emotional and contextual perspective. The diffuse system processes information in several key subcortical sensory centers.

The ability to identify sounds and localize them in space is critical to our survival. Whether the hunter will catch his prey or become the prey, depends on precise determination of both the direction and distance of a sound source. Accurate sound perception and auditory space localization are also essential for the perception of organized tonal patterns found in the speaking voice and in music. The two functions of sound perception and spatial localization (what and where) begin processing interactively in the bilateral cochlear nuclei. The cochlear nuclei are differentiated into the dorsal nucleus for analysis of the tonal properties of sound and the ventral nucleus that identifies where sound is located. Tonal patterns help us to discriminate between different sounds. For example, we are able to differentiate the tonal pattern of a lion's roar from that of a chirping bird. The ventral nucleus tells us where sound is by analyzing the time of arrival and the intensity (volume) of the sound.

Since sound does not arrive at the two ears at the same time, this time interval difference must be analyzed and compared in order to locate sounds in space and to encode spatial relationships. Sixty percent of the nerve fibers from each ear cross over to the contralateral side of the brain stem to facilitate comparison of auditory input. The superior olivary complex, because it receives many of these crossed auditory fibers, facilitates the two ventral auditory nuclei's ability to identify where something is by comparing the difference in arrival time with the variance in the intensity of the sound between the two ears. There are important clues that allow you to determine the precise location of the sound source. A sound that is behind you and slightly to the left will reach your left ear first (arrival time difference) and be slightly louder (more intense) in the left ear than the right ear.

Auditory signals are then passed on from the superior olivary complex to the inferior colliculus where both tonal and spatial information from our sound world is integrated with information from our body maps (body scheme). Integration of this information allows us to detect and localize sounds as we move through space. The inferior colliculus is crucial in the orienting response, preparing the body motorically and physiologically for action. The inferior colliculus accomplishes this goal through its connections with over twenty percent of the brain. Many of these connections are with the vestibular related structures because of its critical influence on gaze stabilization during movement, muscle tone, posture and balance and orientation of the body in time and space.

Another important auditory connection is made with the superior colliculus, an important visual processing center for eye movement control and movement detection for survival. The superior colliculus receives information from every sensory system, integrating it into comprehensive body mapping, auditory spatial mapping and visual spatial mapping of the total environment. Working together the inferior and superior colliculi integrate sounds, sights and movements for the purpose of maintaining alert orientation and adaptive behavior in an ever changing environment. Ayres (1972) referred to the vital role of these centers in sensory integrative processing because of their critical task of alerting and orienting the individual within their environment.

The next relay station is the medial geniculate nucleus of the thalamus. Here meaningful sound signals are sharpened while noise is dampened. This process begins as soon as sounds are funneled in the outer ear and is further refined at every stage along the way. This modulation enhances the critical features of the signal into the foreground for sharper focus, laying the foundation for the development of auditory figure ground skills. The medial geniculate nucleus is not fully myelinated until about 10 years of age.

Prior to sending signals on to the cortex, all of the subcortical relay stations play an important part in sharpening the edges of a sound by comparing and contrasting the difference between higher and lower tones. At each of these relay stations the auditory messages become clearer and more precise. Cells are stimulated throughout the duration of sound emission at the lowest level. At higher levels, cells fire only at the beginning and end of a tone so as to discriminate the salient features of the soundscape.

The primary auditory cortex responds selectively to particular frequencies, similar to the auditory nerve and several of the relay points along the afferent auditory pathway. Just as sounds are received in an orderly fashion along the basilar membrane, the cortical cells are arranged in an orderly fashion from low to high tones. The temporal cortex is concerned with analyzing the temporal spatial as well as the tonal properties of sound, utilizing a systematic arrangement referred to as tonotopic organization. Cells of similar frequencies (tones) are placed next to each other. These cells are layered on top of another group of cells that are organized according to the temporal spatial aspects of sound. Following analysis of the tonal and temporal spatial aspects of sound, further processing unfolds in the association area of the posterior parietal lobe.

There is bilaterality of the auditory projections throughout the central nervous system from the ears to the cortex because of unilateral and contralateral afferent projections that support the integration of the sound information coming from each ear. Sound received in one ear produces greater activity in the opposite hemisphere because of a preponderance of contralateral fiber projections. Each hemisphere has a specialized orientation in the process of analyzing sound and executing cognitive auditory processing endeavors. The left hemisphere is responsible for analyzing the temporal and sequential patterns of sound while the right hemisphere is concerned with the spatial properties of sound. Learning language and related academic skills entails left hemisphere specialization skills that include reception and expression of language symbols, rhythm, ideation and sequencing. It also depends on right hemisphere contribution of the larger spatial context and construction, melody and emotional intonation. Both ways of processing sound are critical for learning, memory, creative thought and expression.

Central Processing of
Vestibular-Auditory Information

Just as sound and movement travel along well differentiated pathways, they concurrently interface with a more diffuse processing system. The eighth cranial nerve, for example has direct and indirect connections with major processing centers including the reticular formation, the limbic system and the autonomic nervous system.

Reticular Formation

The reticular formation is located deep within the brain stem and receives diffuse sensory input from multiple structures. It is a very old part of the brain concerned with basic survival issues. The major function of the reticular formation is to control states of consciousness ranging from asleep to alert and to generate inherent rhythms e.g. circadian rhythms. It plays a major role in setting cell thresholds. While it enhances some features of sensation it, dampens others. The reticular formation acts as a filter, allowing conscious awareness of some sensations and screening others out. This screening process is based on factors of novelty and intensity. Both ascending and descending pathways (to the cortex and to the spinal cord) contribute to the moment-to-moment modulation of incoming signals. Consider what happens when you hear a loud bang (both novel and intense): your body may startle, increasing extensor tone throughout your body as you turn your head and search for the offending noise (Moore, J. C. & Farber, S. D., 1990).

Limbic System

The limbic system is often considered the emotional brain. It is tied to basic drives and survival behaviors as well as to the perception and expression of emotion. Through its extensive connections to many neural structures and pathways and its role in emotional tone, limbic responses have a profound impact on all aspects of our behavior. The limbic system coordinates several important centers that process sensation. It interfaces with brain stem centers to create an appropriate balance between emotions and alertness. Through connections with the forebrain, it maintains a balance between rational and emotional reactivity. The long term storage of important memories is laid down through the hippocampus and amygdala. They attach affective meaning to memories, thereby enhancing storage and retrieval. The hypothalamus, another important limbic structure, is the route through which autonomic responses are activated to reflect a person's emotional state. It is much easier to remember even the smallest of details around events that are emotionally charged (such as the death of a loved one or a national disaster like the 9/11/01 terrorist attacks).

Autonomic Nervous System

The autonomic nervous system (ANS) is our involuntary nervous system that responds to external stress and regulates our body functions, such as heart rate, respiration, digestion, as well as bowel and bladder function. The autonomic nervous system is divided into two branches, the sympathetic nervous system (SNS) and the parasympathetic nervous system (PNS). These neural systems originate in the brainstem and contribute the regulation of a variety of target organs, including:

• the eyes	• lacrimal glands	• salivary gland
• sweat glands	• blood vessels	• heart
• lungs	• trachea	• lungs
• stomach	• kidney	• pancreas
• intestines	• external genitalia	• bladder

The PNS and SNS work together to maintain these end organs within an optimal range of function. In general the SNS branch increases activity level and directs energy outward to deal with challenges outside the body. The PNS promotes functions of growth and restoration through energy conservation.

The SNS and PNS branches' effects are antagonistic. The SNS dilates the pupils, increases heart rate, inhibits intestinal movement and contracts vesical and rectal sphincters. The PNS constricts the pupils, decreases heart rate, increases gut motility and relaxes the vesical and rectal sphincters. When the system is biased toward parasympathetic, one becomes more relaxed and internally focused, promoting growth and restoration.

The SNS, on the other hand, is most often associated with the fight/flight/fright response. It is also involved in preparing for action in response to external demands and environmental challenges. The SNS quickly mobilizes the existing reserve of the body. When this system is dominant, the pupils dilate, the heart rate increases and there is a concomitant increase in blood pressure. The blood is drained from the intestines to increase the availability of blood flow to the skeletal muscles, lungs, heart and brain. Peristalsis and elimination are also inhibited.

The SNS and PNS coordinate their responses according to internal and external demands. The PNS is modulated by internal change in the viscera. The SNS is primarily activated by exteroceptive impulses in response to changes in the external environment.

The ability of these two systems to coordinate their actions has a strong affect on attention and behavior. This can be seen in their coordinated efforts during the orienting response. When something novel is introduced into the environment there is an initial increase in heart rate and respiration. This is followed by a decrease in respiration rate and, in turn, a suppression of heart rate. Steve Porges (1964), in his work with vagal tone, found that individual differences with inhibitory control of heart rate (through coupling heart rate with respiration) parallel the differences in ability to attend. In his work with disregulated infants, he showed that a reduction of respiratory activity and heart rate variability went hand in hand with longer 'on task' behavior.

Polyvagal Theory

Extensive work on the neural regulation of the autonomic nervous system led Porges to propose the Polyvagal Theory. His theory explores the relationship between the autonomic nervous system and the social engagement process. He describes three global stages that the ANS undergoes in its evolutionary development and their relationship to behavioral strategies. The first stage of development is the most primitive function of the unmyelinated vagus nerve that regulates the gut. This portion of the vagus nerve promotes digestion and peristalsis and responds to threat with immobilizing and freezing behaviors including depression of metabolic activity.

The second stage of development involves two simultaneous SNS actions. These are increasing metabolic output (increase in heart rate, respiration and blood flow to the limbs) and concomitant depression of the visceral vagus (inhibition of gut function) to foster the mobilization behavior for fight or flight.

Stage three is the myelinated vagus which can rapidly regulate cardiac output for the purposes of promoting engagement or disengagement with the environment. This most recent evolutionary development is unique to mammals. The older unmyelinated system regulates the gut while the newer myelinated vagus influences the heart. This newer, vagus system serves to dampen sympathetic reaction to stress and promote self regulation and sustained attention (DeGangi & Porges, 1991). It takes an active role in coupling heart rate and respiration to functionally slow the heart rate to achieve and maintain a calm state. The myelinated portion of the vagus nerve originates in the lower brain stem where it is neuroanatomically connected to the muscles of the middle ear, jaw, facial expression and the muscles responsible for vocalization and head turning (CNs VII, V, IX & XII, respectively). This lower portion of the brainstem is under the control of the frontal cortex during facial expression and vocal interactions that lead to initiation and sustenance of social interaction. Porges (2001) contends that in addition these connections being functional, they have evolved together for the purposes of promoting social behaviors and communication.

During times of stress, according to Polyvagal Theory, the cortical control of the newly evolved, myelinated vagus and neurophysiological supports for social engagement are subjugated to the older more primitive vagal system. The more primitive, unmyelinated system is driven by subcortical structures that regulate metabolic resources to expend energy for fight and flight behavior by immobilizing or shutting down to conserve energy. Therefore, under conditions of perceived threat in the environment, the mechanisms that promote social behavior will disintegrate. The middle ear mechanism, playing a key role in listening, will be less effective in focusing on human voice and revert to more primitive focus on the low frequency dominated background. Since it shares neural structures with the myelinated vagus and biological substrates of social engagement and communication, the middle ear is a critical component of these functions. As such, it offers a therapeutic avenue for making significant changes in listening, verbal and non-verbal communication and other aspects of social-emotional relatedness (Porges, et al 1997).

Neurochemical Possibilities

The differentiated central processing of sound and movement through the above mentioned circuits, although less clearly defined, has an associated chemistry that is involved in attention, memory, motivation and learning. The chemical messengers from the autonomic nervous system, reticular formation and the limbic system interact through complex circuitry to allow us to assign meaning and value to a given sensory experience. Cool (1991) discusses the importance of the biogenic amines (epinephrine, norepinephrine, histamine, dopamine and serotonin) as the key chemistry in assigning "meaning and purpose" to any sensorimotor event. The biogenic amines are a class of neurotransmitters that impact countless targets throughout the nervous system. They are associated with the reticular activating system and function in arousal, alerting, attention, emotion and learning. They have a modulating affect within the nervous system either "waking up for action" or "relaxing for rest" (Farber & Cool, 1990).

Cool also points out the role of norepinephrine, highly associated with emotion, as a key ingredient in neuroplasticity. "Norepinephrine inputs to the cerebral cortex initiate the complex cellular process that allows new synapses to form or modify." This process provides "the key to nervous system development, organization, learning, memory and reorganization after perturbation," (Cool, 1990). The amount of emotion attached to any given event will have a direct impact on the level of chemistry mobilized to prepare the cortex for learning and memory.

In her book, *The Molecules of Emotion*, Candice Pert (1997) also emphasizes the important role of emotion in human function. She describes a class of small molecules that are found in the brain, the body and the immune and endocrine system. These small molecules travel in the fluid systems in the body and bind these systems together. Pert likens these molecules to a mobile brain through which the neural, hormonal, gastrointestinal and immune systems communicate and exchange information. These neuropeptides are the substrates of emotion that dictate where to attend. They signal the level of importance and help to direct attention and set up the most appropriate set of behaviors for adaptation. The receptors are not stagnant, shifting according to the circumstance.

Of all the brain systems, the neuropeptides are found in greatest abundance in the autonomic nervous system. Eighty to eighty-five percent of those are found in the limbic system. Another nodal point or hot spot which contains a high percentage of the neuropeptides is the inferior colliculus which is responsible for the orienting response. It is a major processing center for orientation to sound and connecting sounds with movement.

What is meaningful and purposeful will always relate to the 'molecules of emotion.' Emotion sustains our attention. Emotion is important because it always accompanies attention, learning and memory. A person's emotional response marks importance and signals change. An elevation in emotional tone seems to be one of the key signals that we are making change.

Characteristics of Sound

Sound is vibratory energy that takes the form of waves. These waves are measured in units of rate of vibration (cycles per second) or frequency. High pitched sounds vibrate fast with a high frequency. Low pitched sounds vibrate slowly with a low frequency. Sounds up to about 16 Hz are perceived as a rhythm and are sensed as a pulsating movement by the 'ear of the body' (Madaule, 1993), the vestibular system. There is a seamless transition between movement, rhythm and sound. The transition from what is perceived as a movement in the form of rhythm to what is perceived as a tone happens somewhere between 16 - 50 Hz. Therefore low pitched sounds are often associated with movement. Low sound often directs the body to move, both for protection and exploration. Low sounds in nature, such as thunder and earthquakes, signal danger and warn us to move. Rhythm provides a structure for movement, telling us how to move through time and space.

The lower frequencies, along with being closely related to movement and rhythm, also provide information about the background or the space in which they are generated. Sounds below 300 Hz (example: lawn mowers, trucks) have very little directional information, they often fill the background with a low hum but they are hard to locate. The brain is best able to localize sounds in space in the 500 to 1,500 Hz range. Many of the vowel sounds are in this range. Vowels tend to signal us that someone is speaking, assisting us to locate the speaker in space. Low frequency sounds tend to be multidirectional. They fan out in all directions like a floodlight, filling the space in which they are emitted. Low frequency sounds take more energy to generate, are transmitted more easily and travel greater distances. For this reason, background sounds tend to be low and muffled. Lower sounds tend to overpower higher tones.

High frequency sounds are more difficult to transmit than low frequency sounds. Higher frequency sounds perceived from a distance are indistinct (one can notice the difference within two to five feet). Higher pitched sounds are best perceived up close and for this reason they tend to create the foreground.

Higher frequency sounds are unidirectional, meaning that they move in more of a straight line from the sound source, more like a flashlight (Madaule, 2000). High tones provide information regarding the direction and distance of the sound source. They carry the more detailed content and distinguishing characteristics of sounds that make up the foreground. The closer a voice is the better one is able to perceive it. This is not just a matter of volume. A person speaking on a loud speaker may be heard from hundreds of feet away but not understood until one is much closer. It is more a matter of the physical properties of higher frequency sounds. Nature alerts us to what is most important by preserving the detailed information in higher pitched sounds (Steinbach, 1997).

The human ear is much more sensitive and able to discriminate sounds in the mid-frequency range. It is the most sensitive to pitch changes between 1,000 and 3,000 Hz. The range from 2,000 to 4,000 Hz is the frequency range in which the key sounds S, Z, Sh and the P, B, K, D are captured (Schiffman, 1996). These sounds are critical for understanding speech and giving words clarity and definition (Wilson, 1991).

Sounds above 4,000 Hz carry more subtle, detailed information about the individual qualities of the source of the sound and the space in which it is emitted. This part of the sound spectrum adds timbre or color to the sound. It is the part of the sound spectrum that adds interest and variety to sounds, helping to capture and maintain our interest. Most computer-generated voices do not have many of these upper frequencies and their patterns are more simple. For the typical listener, this makes them difficult to listen to for an extended period of time. The ability to detect sounds in the upper frequency range varies. While the newborn can detect sounds up to 20,000 to 25,000 Hz, the average adult can detect upper frequencies ranges only to 12,000 to 15,000 Hz.

Even though we are not consciously aware of many of the upper frequencies they do have an impact on us. One study conducted by Ingo Steinbach at the University of Dortmund in Germany showed that a group of students could not respond to frequencies above 15,000 to 16,000 Hz, when tested with standard audiometric measures (Steinbach, 1997). However, they were able to detect changes in music that had frequencies above 16,000 Hz filtered out. We typically don't consciously detect these frequencies when made by themselves, but they do have an impact on us as part of complex sound matrices known as harmonics (to be addressed later).

The volume or intensity of a particular sound is measured in decibels. In the decibel scale the faintest sound one can hear is labeled zero decibels (0dB), which is considered the normal threshold for human hearing. The decibel scales are logarithmic so that an increase of 10 dB represents a tenfold increase in intensity; 20 dB represents 100 fold and 30 dB represents a 1,000 fold increase. The entire range of sound from the threshold to the loudest sound is 150 dB. The difference in energy would be from one to a quadrillion. This makes the human ear equipped to be one of the most discriminating senses, especially as a distance receptor.

The ear is the most sensitive to high tones that require only a fraction of the energy to sound as loud as a midrange tone. Played softly, a low frequency tone must have ten times the energy of a midrange tone to sound as loud and almost 100 times the energy at high volume. This is one reason why damage to hearing may be caused by listening to music on headphones that contain bass instruments, drums, brass and/or electronic instruments. The lower frequency sounds need to be increased in volume to be perceived with the high sounds. That makes the sounds much too intense to be funneled into delicate human hearing mechanisms. Wearing headphones removes that space and places sounds meant to be felt though the body dangerously close to the eardrum.

Normally we perceive what seems like a single tone when we hear a note sung or played by an instrument. However in nature, sound producing sources don't vibrate at a single frequency. Within any given note there is an entire spectrum of sound. In general, several frequencies vibrate simultaneously, creating a complex sound structure. The individual frequencies are termed 'partials.' The partial having the lowest frequency is called the fundamental frequency or the first harmonic. The fundamental frequency determines the pitch of a complex sound. For example, when a string is plucked, the full-length vibration produces the fundamental frequency. In addition, there are vibrations of shorter lengths, higher frequencies (precise divisions of the strings' length) that are called overtones or harmonics. The relationship of the overtones to the fundamental is an exact mathematical relationship with a strict, orderly structure. In general, all of the overtones are higher in pitch and all are multiples of the fundamental.

These additional sounds, called harmonics (overtones, partials), are responsible for shaping the uniqueness of individual instruments and human voices. The harmonics have a very orderly pattern or structure whereas noise has a disorderly, unpredictable structure. Overtones are mathematical ratios of the first note, or the fundamental. We tend to identify a tone by its lowest and loudest component. In most cases, you cannot distinguish the different individual overtones which make up sounds.

The number and intensity (volume) of the harmonics give sounds their specific tonal qualities (timbre). Different instruments emit and emphasize different harmonics. This is how we can distinguish among instruments when they play the same note. Instruments that produce many harmonics (i.e. guitar, piano) give a fuller, richer sound. Each instrument and voice has its own characteristic overtones which create a unique sound pattern, like a 'fingerprint' for that voice or instrument (Steinbach, 1997).

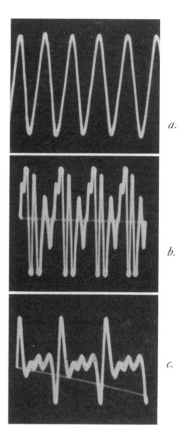

Fig. 2-11.

From Culver, 1956, pg. 103.
a. Tuning fork at 440 Hz; single wave form

b. Clarinet at 440 Hz; fundamental with subsequent overtones.

c. Cornet at 440Hz; fundamental with subsequent overtones.

The number of overtones and the relative intensity gives each sound individual shape and tonal characteristics. It is this shape that is exaggerated in spectral activation.

Overtones are responsible for shaping the sounds that we hear, giving each instrument and voice its unique sound qualities. If both the piano and flute were to play middle C, they would be virtually indistinguishable from each other should their particular overtone patterns be filtered out.

In addition to differentiating one sound from another, the individual volume distribution of the overtones also transmits subtle detailed information content. The individual volume distribution shapes the sounds and is called the envelope shaped curve.

Our attention is triggered by the parts of the sound spectrum where the sounds are the most intensive or stressed. The frequency content of the sounds stays the same. However, when something is important, the amplitude (volume) of the overtones change. The shape of the sound, with increases in the volume or amplitude of the individual overtones, indicates importance and attaches interest and meaning to sounds. Increasing the upper tones stimulates human alertness. When many high tones reach the ears, they signal it to listen carefully— to pay attention. Changing the shape of the sound changes the meaning of the sound. We know that we can say the same word or phrase several different ways, each time drastically changing the meaning. It is this natural phenomenon that Steinbach captures in all recordings and intensifies in the process he terms 'spectral activation.'

The overtones not only help us distinguish one instrument from another, they carry the more detailed inferences about location, direction and their overall importance in any particular group of sounds. These finer details and meanings of sounds are found in the harmonic structure and the individual volume distribution of the harmonics.

Our brain is designed to find and create order. It can easily make sense from structured harmonic patterns. If the distance between the overtones were uneven the brain would need to work much harder. Patterns are easier to remember. For noise, overtones are unclear because there is no pattern. As a result, we can appreciate how draining, frightening and/or disruptive noise can be to us.

References/Suggested Readings

Ayres, A. J. (1972). *Sensory integration and learning disorders.* Los Angeles: Western Psychological Services.

Ayres, A. J. (1979). *Sensory integration and the child.* Los Angeles: Western Psychological Services.

Barr, M. L. (1979). *The human nervous system.* New York: Harper & Row.

Bennett, K. E. & Haggard, M. P. (1999). Behavior and cognitive outcomes from middle ear disease. *Archives of Disability in Children,* 80, 28-35.

Borg, E. & Counter, S. A. (1989, Aug). The middle ear muscles. *Scientific American,* 74-80.

Brewer, C. & Campbell, D. (1991). *Rhythms of learning.* Tucson, AZ: Zephyr Press.

Cohen, H. & Keshner, E. A. (1989). Current concepts of the vestibular system reviewed: Part 1, The role of the vestibulospinal system in postural control. *The American Journal of Occupational Therapy, 43* (5), 320-330.

Cohen, H. & Keshner, E. A. (1989). Current concepts of the vestibular system reviewed: Part 2, Visual/vestibular intervention and spatial orientation. *The American Journal of Occupational Therapy, 43* (5), 331-338.

Condon, W. & Sander, L. (1974). Neonate movement is synchronized with adult speech: Interactional participation and language acquisition. *Science, 11* (99), 1.

Condon, W. S. (1975). Multiple response to sound in dysfunctional children. *Journal of Autism and Childhood Schizophrenia,* 5, 37-56.

Cool, S. J. (1987). A view from 'outside:' Sensory integration and developmental neurobiology. *AOTA Sensory Integration Special Interest Section Newsletter, 10* (2), 2-3.

Cool, S. J. (1992) *Pain, plasticity, allergies and behavior: Neurobiological discoveries of 1991.* Workshop presentation. Minneapolis, MN.

Cool, S. J. (2001). *Full inclusion: Vision and hearing in sensory integration practice.* Workshop presentation. New York, NY.

Culver, C. A. (1956). *Musical acoustics.* New York: McGraw-Hill.

DeGangi, G.A., & Porges, S.W. (1991). Attention/alertness/arousal. In C. B. Royeen (Ed.) *AOTA Self Study Series*, Rockville, MD: The American Occupational Therapy Association.

Eckman, P. & Friesen, W. V. (1967). Head and body cues in the judgment of emotion: A reformulation. *Perceptual and Motor Skills, 24,* 711-724.

Eckman, P., Levenson, R. W., & Friesen, W. V. (1983). Autonomic nervous system activity distinguishes among emotions. *Science, 221,* 1208-1210.

Elliot, L. (1999). *What's going on in there? How the brain and mind develop in the first five years of life.* New York: Bantam Books.

Farber, S., & Huss, A. J. (1974). *Sensorimotor evaluation and treatment procedures.* Indianapolis, IN: Indiana University, Indianapolis Medical Center.

Farber, S. D., & Cool, S. J. (1990). Functional neurochemistry. In C. B. Royeen (Ed.), *Neuroscience foundations of human performance* (Chapter 4). Rockville, MD: American Occupational Therapy Association.

Greenspan, S., & Porges, S. (1983, Nov-Dec). Psychopathology in infancy and early childhood: Clinical perspectives on the organization of sensory and affective-thematic experience. *Child Development.*

Jourdain, R. (1997). *Music, the brain and ecstacy: How music captures our imagination.* New York: Avon Books.

Kandel, E. R., Schwartz, J. H., & Jessell, T. M. (2000). *Principles of neural science* (4th ed.). New York: McGraw-Hill Companies, Inc.

MacLean, P. D. (1977). The triune brain in conflict. *Psychotherapy and Psychosomatics, 28,* 201-220.

Madaule, P. (1993). *When listening comes alive.* Ontario: Moulin Publishing.

Madaule, P. (2000). *Listening fitness™ trainers manual.* Toronto: The Listening Centre.

Montgomery, P. C. (1981). *The vestibular system: An annotated bibliography.* Torrance, CA: Sensory Integration International.

Moore, J. C. (1972). Cranial nerves and their importance in current rehabilitation techniques. In A. Henderson & J. Coryell (Eds.), *The body senses and perceptual deficits.* Boston, MA: School of Occupational Therapy, Boston University.

Moore, J. C., & Farber, S.D. (1990). Systemic neuroanatomy. In Royeen, C. B. (Ed.), *AOTA self study series.* Rockville, MD: The American Occupational Therapy Association.

Moore, J. C. (1994). The functional components of the nervous system: Part I. *Sensory Integration Quarterly, XXII* (3), 1-7.

Moore, J. C. (1995). The functional components of the nervous system: Part II. *Sensory Integration Quarterly, XXII* (4), 1-9.

Morris, S. E. & Klein, M. D. (1987). *Pre-feeding skills.* Tucson, AZ: Therapy Skill Builders.

Moyers, B. (1993). *Healing and the mind.* New York: Doubleday.

Netter, F. H. (1986). *Ciba collection of medical illustrations: Vol 1, Nervous System: Part I, Anatomy and physiology.* Ciba Pharmaceutical, Inc.

Oetter, P., Laurel, M. K., & Cool, S. J. (1990). Sensorimotor foundations of communication. In C. B. Royeen (Ed.), *AOTA Self Study Series.* Rockville, MD: The American Occupational Therapy Association.

Oetter, P., Richter, E. & Frick, S. (1995). *MORE: Integrating the mouth with sensory and postural functions, 2nd Edition.* Hugo, MN: PDP Press, Inc.

Pert, C. (1997). *Molecules of emotion.* New York: Scribner Publishing.

Porges, S. W. (1964). Physiological correlates of attention: A core process underlying learning disorders. *Pediatric Clinics of North America, 31* (2).

Porges, S. W. (1995). Orienting in a defensive world: Mammalian modifications of our evolutionary heritage. A Polyvagal Theory. *Psychophysiology, 32,* 301-318.

Porges, S. W., Doussard-Roosevelt, J. A., Portales, A. L., & Greenspan, S. I. (1996). Infant regulation of the vagal "brake" predicts child behavior problems: A psychobiological model of social behavior. *Developmental Psychobiology, 29,* 697-712.

Porges, S. W., Bazhenova, O., Carlson, N., Apparies, R., & Roa, P. (1997, November). *New interventions to enhance language, reading and learning.* Presentation. Washington, DC.

Porges, S. W. (2001). The polyvagal theory: phylogenetic substrates of a social nervous system. *International Journal of Psychophysiology, 42* (2), 29-52.

Pribram, K. H., & McGuinness, D. (1975). Arousal, activation and efforts in the control of attention. *Psychological Review, 32,* 116-149.

Schiffman, H. R. (1996). *Sensation and perception: An integrated approach* (4th ed.). New York: John Wiley & Sons, Inc.

Steinbach, I. (1997). *SAMONAS sound therapy: The way to health through sound.* Germany: Techau Verlag.

Steinbach, I. (1999). *SAMONAS sound therapy handbook.* Germany: Techau Verlag.

Steinbach, I. (2000). www.samonas.com

Steinbach, I. (2001). *SAMONAS core training.* Workshop presentation, Madison, WI.

Tallal, P., Miller, S., Fitch, R. (1993). Neurobiological basis of speech: A case for the preeminence of temporal processing, In: *Temporal information processing in the nervous system: Special reference to dyslexia and dysphasia,* P. Tallal, A. M., Galaburda, R. R., Llinas and C. Von Euler (Eds), Annals of the New York Academy of Sciences, 682, 27-47.

The Senses. (1997, January 13). *U.S. News & World Report,* 52-54.

Trott, M. C., Laurel, M. K., & Windek, S. L. (1993). *SenseAbilities: Understanding sensory integration.* Tucson, AZ: Communication Skill Builders.

Verny, T. (1981). *The secret life of the unborn child.* New York: Dell Publishing.

Wilson, T. (1991). Chant: the healing power of voice and ear. In: *Music: Physician for times to come.* Campbell, ed. Wheaton, IL: Quest.

Guidelines for Therapeutic Listening Programs

3

When designing a Therapeutic Listening program specifically tailored to an individual's needs, there are several factors or variables that must be considered. These variables are: **the music, the manner in which music has been changed or altered, the duration of listening sessions and the frequency of listening sessions.** It is only when these variables are carefully addressed that maximum benefit from a Therapeutic Listening program can occur. Additionally, when benefits do not seem to be occurring, these same variables should be altered until the "best fit" between an individual and a Therapeutic Listening program has been created.

It is important to remember that the ideas shared here are just guidelines; therapists must rely upon their own clinical reasoning skills as they begin to use the sound technology. It can be easy to interpret the guidelines given as rules when beginning to implement Therapeutic Listening programs; however, Therapeutic Listening programs should be based on solid clinical reasoning and not a recipe approach.

Clinical Considerations when Choosing Music

Music has been used as a therapeutic tool since the beginning of civilization. A number of research studies are emerging in the literature that demonstrate the impact of music on the physiological correlates of arousal and emotion, several aspects of motor control, cognitive perceptual skills and learning.

To better understand the impact of music and learn how to clinically reason which music might best support a client's individual treatment needs in a Therapeutic Listening program, it is important to first have a basic understanding of the elements of music and their relative impact on function. Traditionally those who use music to enhance performance focus on five elements: tone, rhythm, melody, harmony and timbre or texture. For our purposes, especially when choosing music from SAMONAS recordings, we will also consider the spatial aspects of the music and the qualities of the recording space.

Musical Elements
Tone

Every note is created by a specific rate of vibration that can have a physical and psychological impact on the individual. Each musical note has a specific quality that has the potential to affect physical and emotional reactions, but one cannot ascribe a specific quality to a note since each individual reacts in subtly different ways. Furthermore, with music, as with all natural sounds, we don't perceive tones individually. In general the lower the tone, the more related its impact is to physical aspects, like body movement, and the more basic its emotional impact. The higher the tone, the more related to higher level, sophisticated processes of emotion, attention and cognition. Contrast the effect of primitive drumming versus a Mozart violin concerto.

Rhythm

Rhythm, a pattern of accentuated beats, is the most fundamental element of music. The most basic *form* of music, common in the music of primitive peoples, consists solely of rhythm. In most musical forms rhythm is used to provide the grid or structure on which musical thoughts are built.

Rhythm provides the time element in any given musical piece. There are two elements in rhythm: meter and tempo. Meter, or the grouping of beats, is a special organization of the time elements that have developed over centuries. The groups are generally in patterns of 2, 3, or 4 equally timed beats, with stress on the first beat of the group. Once the pattern is established the listener can anticipate when notes will begin and end. Meter lends predictability and order to the music.

Tempo is speed (andante, moderato, allegro, etc.). The greater the tempo the greater the emotional tension produced. The tempo of music has a powerful influence on coordinating the physiological rhythms of the body. The rhythm of various bodily functions can be influenced by the tempo of the music by a principle known as entrainment. Entrainment is the process of two rhythms developing the same pulse through proximity to one another. Through entrainment the stronger vibration of one object can cause a less powerful object to synchronize and vibrate at the rate of the stronger object. The sounds and rhythms available in music are very effective entrainment tools. Through sound it is possible to entrain the different rhythms of the body and influence the rhythmical pulsing of electrical brain activity, i.e. marching to a drum beat, or a chant cadence. Entrainment, this locking in step of vibrations, was first described by Dutch scientist, Christian Huygen in 1665. Slower tempos, around 50-70 beats per minute, tend to influence heart rate, respiration and suck/swallow/breathe rhythms.

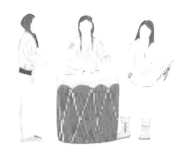

Entrainment is the process of two rhythms developing the same pulse through proximity to one another. Through entrainment the stronger vibration of one object can cause a less powerful object to synchronize and vibrate at the rate of the stronger object. The sounds and rhythms available in music are very effective entrainment tools.

Through the principles of entrainment, music can also have a powerful impact on the electrical activity of the brain. The patterns, know as brain waves, cycle at different rates, creating a variety of patterns that are closely related to states of alertness. For example the music of Mozart tends to increase the electrical firing in the faster cycles of the beta range. Beta is related to focused attention, organized thought and behavior patterns and the quick ability to react to external stimuli. In contrast, the slower movements of Baroque music and *Gregorian Chant* have been shown to increase the activity in a slightly slower firing pattern know as alpha. Alpha corresponds to the quiet alert state, one of the best states for openness and receptivity to new learning as well as retaining and integrating information that is learned. Interestingly this same tempo in Baroque music has been shown to entrain sucking rate in infants (Morris, 1982).

The tempo of the music chosen can also impact our sense of time. The speed of the music chosen can either speed up or slow down alertness, quality and time of response. Music of the Classical and Baroque periods tends to promote more organized physiological and behavioral responses (i.e. sucking, chewing, respiratory patterns with movement; gait; movement patterns, etc.).

Rhythm is the physical aspect of music. Of all the elements in music, it has the most intense and immediate influence on the body. As discussed in several studies by Michael Thaut, Ph.D., a researcher in the field of music therapy, rhythm has a specific effect on the motor systems of the body (Thaut, Schleiffers, & Davis, 1991). His work has investigated how the auditory system processes information in relationship to the sensory and motor systems of the body. In studying the interaction of the auditory and motor systems, using standard measures of muscle activity such as EMG studies, Thaut demonstrated that rhythmic auditory stimulation can increase the duration of muscle activity, improve muscular endurance and increase the coordination and cocontraction patterns of opposing muscle groups.

Melody

Melody is a combination of rhythms, tones and accents that produce musical units or wholes. These elements form a particular pattern of sound and a system of relationships between notes. Music elements of fixed pitch, duration and accent provide the anchor points among which a brain can discern relationships and interrelationships. Melody is the subject matter of a musical piece. It unfolds in a horizontal line over time giving us the horizontal element of space and forward progression.

Melodies, a synthesis of various musical factors, can create physical sensations that may invite body movement, move the listener emotionally, or stimulate visualization, memories or

> *Brain Wave Frequencies:*
>
> *Delta - (slow firing) deep dreamless, sleep, very deep breathing, slow heart rate, cool body temperature*
>
> *Theta - (mainly in temporal & parietal regions of the brain) unconscious sleep state, deep meditation, deep creative dreams, deep creative thought*
>
> *Alpha - (brain idle or midpoint, Cool, 1999) relaxation, daydreaming, creative imagination, connection to subconscious, information synthesis, first assimilation, integrated learning states*
>
> *Beta - (most commonly recorded in frontal and parietal lobe) logical thought processing, analysis, active, organizational skills, productivity, attention, external focus*
>
> *High Beta - anxiety, anger, short/shallow breathing*

thought patterns. These elements in music can be used as a tool to direct and support the listener in physical, emotional and cognitive performance.

Harmony

Harmony is created when notes are sounded together, either simultaneously or successively, and blend with each other to form chords. According to the respective rates of vibration of these sounds, the result is either a harmonious blending or jarring discord. Either way, harmony has an impact on the emotional tone and the feeling of depth in a musical selection. Different intervals, chords or combinations are joined to evoke emotions. Harmony also adds a vertical dimension to music. As the tones are stacked on top of each other they create the dimension of depth.

Timbre (tone color or quality)/ Texture

The nature and structure of various musical instruments including the human voice give each sound pattern a special quality that is easily recognized because it evokes different physical and emotional responses. Each individual experiences the different quality of the trumpet, violin or flute.

Texture is the overall impression a piece of music creates, the actual feel of the sound experience. Texture is not based on a single definable element but on several factors such as the instruments played, the dynamic range (loud to soft) and the relative complexity of the music. Music has the power to create a strong physical impression. For example, the music of Mozart gives the overall impression of order, elegance and balance.

Space

The element of the music or the sound recorded can add to our perception of spaciousness in a recording. Music with slower tempos and environmental recordings contain more space between the tones. The spatial dimensions of music may also be present in the depth felt with rich harmonic structures. Ambient, nature sounds recordings tend to give one a sense of spaciousness.

Ingo Steinbach, the creator of SAMONAS, takes this idea a step further when he creates a recording. He has developed a highly specialized process for selecting music and nature sounds. He also takes the qualities of the recording space into account. Most of his music has been recorded in places that have superior acoustic properties, such as various chapels, cathedrals and churches throughout Europe. Care is taken during every step of the recording process to accurately reproduce the spatial qualities of the sound and preserve the high frequencies up to 20,000 Hz. This attention to detail and the spatial elements of music and the recording space are unique to the SAMONAS Sound Therapy.

To be able to perceive space and accurately discriminate sounds within a given space one must first be able to sense one's place in the surrounding space. This is accomplished in all SAMONAS recordings by a specially designed microphone arrangement that allows the recording to be perceived from the 'reference point of the listener' as well as giving the most accurate image of the space. Including the spatial aspect in sounds has a profound impact on spatial skill since the auditory, along with the vestibular sense, gives us our most basic spatial orienting skills. The development and the refinement of higher level spatial skill is dependent on accurate interpretation of our body or inward sense of space in coordination with our outward extension of this perception of the external environment.

The space reflected in the recording, along with the characteristics of the music, must also fit the needs of the client. For example the client who has very poor awareness of space may benefit from '*Sounds of Nature*' (a SAMONAS recording, p. 3-25). The space in this recording is vast and is one of the major elements in this recording. The sounds of the birds create a simple pattern and sound structure. There is no melody or rhythmic structure. In contrast, the space in '*Live in Catalunya*' (p. 3-23) is large with well-defined limits and the music is quite complex with multiple layers. The first recording is used in most beginning listening protocols to enhance perception of space while the second is used in more selective and individualized protocols to refine skill at a higher level.

Instrumentation

Instrumentation of the recording is as important as the composition of the music selected. The frequency range within which an instrument plays is one consideration. Lower frequency sounds give us information about how to move our bodies. Middle frequency sounds are in the range of human speech and can help to sharpen our communicative skills. Higher frequency sounds help captivate our attention and invite and engage us outward; more detailed, discriminative information is carried in the high frequencies.

The manner in which an instrument is played is also important. Some instruments are "body" instruments (i.e. guitar, cello); they are played close to the body and have a characteristic warmth and resonance to their tonal qualities. As is easily imaginable, they provide information to our bodies and are typically 'grounding' and 'centering.' "Structure" instruments are played away from the body (i.e. harp, piano). As their name suggests they help provide structure and organization; they often delineate time. Finally, "breath" instruments (i.e. flute, clarinet) often trigger attention outward and may help facilitate respiratory and speech patterns.

Percussion

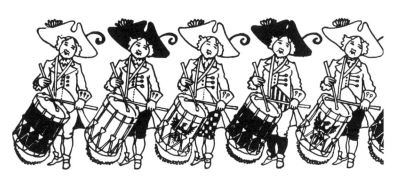

Percussion instruments provide the rhythmic basis to music. They create the bass line, setting a regular, throbbing pulse beneath the other instruments. The drum is the oldest instrument on earth and seems to set up pulses that duplicate heart rate and brain waves. It also activates and organizes the motor systems of the body. *Unless music with a strong bass line has been filtered or modulated it is not appropriate for use over headphones.* The strong pulsing of the rhythm instruments is meant to be experienced in a large space that is absent when music is played through headphones and may damage the ear (even at low volumes and especially at high volumes).

Piano

The piano is considered a structure instrument. The striking of the keys provides clear demarcation of time. The broad frequency range through which a piano plays can provide both a background beat or rhythm around which to organize and a melodic line to captivate attention.

Harp

The harp is another structure instrument. The strings can be plucked to mark time or strummed to create greater fluidity. Like the piano, it plays through a broad frequency range.

Guitar

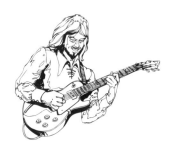

The guitar is considered to be a body instrument as it is played close to the body. It typically has more resonance or warmth to its tone than a harp or piano might. It often creates a grounding or connecting presence in the music. Used in combination with a breath instrument such as a flute, the guitar often provides the foundation for the body upon which the flute then invites attention and focus outward.

Strings (Bass, Cello, Violin)

String instruments are found in chamber music recordings. They are also considered body instruments. The cello, in par-

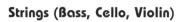

ticular, is enveloped by the musician's body when played; its shape mirrors the human shape. The frequency range in which each of the string instruments plays varies. The bass and cello have a lower frequency range which is generally organizing for the body. The violin is very rich in higher frequency sounds. Its multiple, subtle variations in sound patterns generates a harmonic structure that is most like the subtle variations of the human voice. For that reason the violin is often prominent in the poignant sections of movie sound tracks.

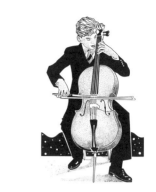

Wind or "Breath" Instruments (Clarinet, Flute)

Wind or breath instruments are related to the body in a different manner than the instruments previously discussed. Their frequency range is narrowly related to the human voice. The clarinet has a broader frequency range than the flute. Because the flute is typically made of metal while the clarinet is typically made of wood (and also played with a reed), the flute tends to have a brighter, thinner sound while the clarinet has more resonance and vibration. The flute's sound pattern is one of the simplest, approaching a pure tone. Its sound is quite transient, requiring one to reach toward the sound thereby capturing attention and focus.

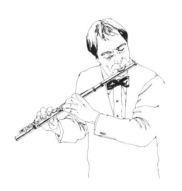

Clearly delineating the desired goals and outcomes attached to treatment and a Therapeutic Listening program will lead to selection of the composition and instrumentation of the music most likely to facilitate those changes.

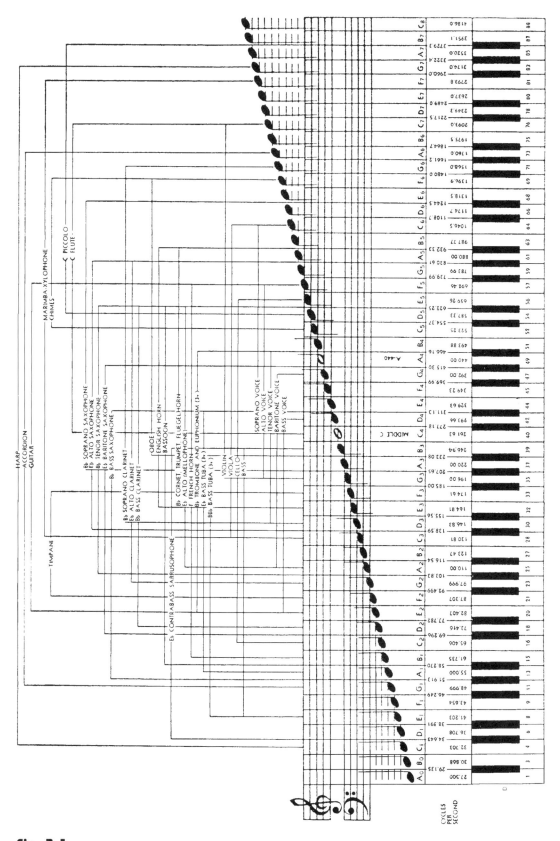

Fig. 3-1

Chart showing the frequency range of voice and various musical instruments. (C. G. Conn, Ltd., out of print)

Listening with the Whole Body

Commercially Available, Non-Modulated Music

There are several commercially available CDs that are frequently used as a therapeutic tool to enhance treatment programs. When choosing music one may consider a number of principles.

♦ Musical selections that are dominated by more lower frequency based instruments (drums) have a strong bass line and clear rhythmic structure that enhances movement based experiences both in the clinic and at home (*Spirit of the Forest; Sacred Spirit Drums*).

♦ Music that pulsates at 50-70 beats per minute will entrain biological rhythms. Consider that *Gregorian Chant*s and the slower movements of Baroque are very useful to accompany therapeutic activities and home programs that address the suck/swallow/breathe synchrony, graded respiration and chewing.

♦ *Sacred Earth Drums* is body oriented and grounding, supporting the biological rhythms inherent in movements such as chewing and walking.

♦ The instrumentation, melodic structure and varied rhythms of *Mozart for Modulation* facilitate higher levels of self regulation.

♦ The basic temporal and spatial characteristics of the compositions and instrumentation chosen for *Mozart Strings Quartet #1* are rich in high frequencies and best suited for promoting higher level academics, communication and emotional expression.

Modulation, Spectral Activation, and Filtering

The music used in Therapeutic Listening programs has been electronically activated to enhance the qualities of the music which then capture and sustain attention and improve listening skills. When designing a personalized listening protocol, it is important to first consider the qualities of the music and instrumentation and then the type and level of modulation or activation that is necessary. Most listening protocols begin with modulated music and move on to add music from the SAMONAS range. SAMONAS adds unique elements that are not found in any other listening protocols, such as a much broader application of the therapeutic elements of music and instrumentation, emphasis on the spatial elements of listening and a variety of levels of intensity through a very sophisticated process of modulation known as spectral activation.

Modulated music

All modulated CDs are processed using an alternating high and low pass filter. The high pass filter allows sounds above 1000 Hz to pass uninterrupted and mutes sounds below 1000 Hz. The low pass filter has the opposite effect muting sounds above 1000 Hz and allowing the sounds below 1000 Hz to pass clearly. This pulsating input appears to create a sharp contrast between the lower and upper ends of the sound frequency. The brain stem

Modulation (in the context of auditory interventions): An alternating high pass/low pass filter is used on the recording. The high pass filter allows the higher frequencies to pass, accentuating the auditory foreground; the low pass filter allows the lower frequencies to pass, emphasizing the auditory background. Modulation facilitates a "gross" contrast between foreground, background, near/far, focus/monitor, listen/take a break. It also provides significant input to the vestibular system and central mechanisms for sensory processing.

For grounding, body awareness and movement exploration within a therapy session or as part of home routines. Listed in order of most grounding to most likely to promote movement.

Speakers only:
Chakra Chants
Sacred Earth Drums
Sacred Spirit Drums
Bakka Beyond
No Worries
Kidz Jamz

The strong rhythms and playful melodies on **Rhythm and Rhyme, Kidz Jamz and No Worries** may be used along with movement oriented treatment sessions as well as to organize behavior at transition times.

Gregorian Chants and the slower movements of **Baroque for Modulation** may be used to enhance suck/swallow/breathe with eating and other related oral motor, respiratory activities.

The rhythmic patterns of **Chakra Chants and Dolphin Dreams** works well for those individuals with very poor awareness of their body and how it is connected with the outside world.

Mozart for Modulation, Mozart Strings I & II, Gregorian Chant, and Rhythm and Rhyme may be used in structured listening programs with headphones to promote attention, focus and self regulation.

Structured listening involves use of headphones and daily listening for a set amount of time for the purpose of enhancing attention. Typical listening times are 20-30 minutes a day - high quality, open ear, circumaural headphones are recommended.

Non-Modulated Music

Vestibular/Body/Posture

Chakra Chants
Sacred Earth Drums
Sacred Spirit Drums
Bakka Beyond - Spirit of the Forest
Dolphin Dreams
Rhythmic Kids' Songs -
No Worries; Rhythm & Rhyme, Kidz Jamz

Self-Regulation/Refined Modulation

Gregorian Chant
Mozart for Modulation
Baroque for Modulation
No Worries
Rhythm & Rhyme

Oral/Respiratory

Baroque for Modulation
Gregorian Chant
Mozart for Modulation
Musical Massage

Communication-Sequencing/Timing

Baroque for Modulation
Mozart for Modulation
No Worries
Rhythm & Rhyme

Language

Baroque for Modulation
Mozart for Modulation
Mozart String Quartets I & II

Expression/Emotionality/Engagement

Baroque for Modulation
Mozart for Modulation
Mozart String Quartets I & II

Academics

Baroque for Modulation
Mozart for Modulation
Mozart String Quartets I & II

Fig. 3-2

modulates sound in much the same manner, enhancing the contrast between the high and low sounds and sending only the stops and starts of the sound up to the cortex for further analysis (Jourdain, 1997). Thus, the rhythmic, pulsing input appears to trigger important sensory integrative centers in the brain stem for basic sensorimotor modulation and sensorimotor integration.

The use of modulated music also appears to train the listener's ear to attend to the higher frequencies. The higher frequencies automatically capture attention since these are the frequencies contained in language, music and sounds that provide the listener with detailed information. Based on clinical experience, the rhythmic pulsing of the high/low pass filter seems to activate the central mechanisms in the vestibular system and concomitant subcortical centers for posture and sensory processing. The alternation between the high and low frequency content activates the middle ear mechanism to contract for focus on higher sounds which are close and relax to monitor the ambient auditory surround for anything which may trigger a need to shift of focus. This ability is a skill needed for adequate perception of near and far sounds as well as figure ground perception. Listening is a skill that can be tuned in and out.

The ability to discriminate and focus on the higher sounds is accomplished at many levels of the ear and brain. The middle ear is responsible for the neuromuscular control of this ability to focus. The contraction of the stapedius dampens the lower frequencies and improves the perception of the higher frequencies. The stapedius is a skeletal muscle subject to the effects of low muscle tone and affected by chronic ear infections. If it is not able to grade contraction through its full range with strength, this focusing ability and all outcomes related to the subcortical processing of sound will be hampered. Modulated music appears to act at this level activating, training and fine tuning the function of the stapedius and its resultant control mechanisms within the brain stem. Fine tuning this function clinically appears to improve sensory modulation and integration and allows the listener to pick up speech in a crowded background, judge the distance, distinguish between sounds in the foreground versus the background as well as setting up the mechanisms of the middle ear so that it can tune sounds in and out at will. All of these functions are at the core of good listening skills.

Sensory Modulation Dysfunction

Disorders in sensory modulation can be seen in difficulties establishing internal rhythms such as an difficulties grading respiratory rate and depth; establishing hunger and thirst patterns (when and how much); sleep/wake cycles (when and how much); activity levels (what the child does when) and in behavioral organization (thinking, emotional responses, memory and organization of postural and motor skills).

On the auditory system...
"Sensory systems of such primal survival significance can be expected to be served by several integrating mechanisms at the brain stem and other subcortical locations. Considerable intersensory integration sufficient to direct a simple adaptive response can also be expected."
(Ayres, p. 71, 1972)

Other parameters that are also associated with sensory modulation difficulties are functional range of arousal states and responsivity to sensation. Sensory modulation difficulties are seen in diverse groups of children and typically include over or underresponsivity to stimuli, unusually high or low fluctuations in activity level, difficulties with transitions or change and problems modulating state and organizing behavior.

Stackhouse and Wilbarger (1998) point out that newer models for describing sensory modulation are emerging in the occupational therapy literature. Past models have discussed sensory reactivity and optimal levels of arousal, however the two concepts have not been considered together in one model. Stackhouse and Wilbarger have proposed the following definition for sensory modulation:

> Sensory modulation is the intake of sensation via typical sensory processing mechanisms such that the degree, intensity and quality of the response is graded to match environmental demand and so that the range of optimal performance/adaptation is maintained.
>
> Difficulties with sensory modulation may present as:
> * Problems grading responses to typical low, or high intensity sensation.
> * Problems attaining or maintaining optimal range of arousal or adaptation in various sensory conditions.
> * Display of defensive response to non-noxious and harmless sensory events. (Wilbarger, 1998, p. 7).

Miller (2001) points out that sensory modulation refers to both physiological and behavioral responses. Through recently documented research, she has shown that the behavioral process for sensory modulation is observable, yet the underlying neurophysiological processes of sensory modulation are not yet empirically proven.

> Miller and others (2001) describe the behavioral manifestations of sensory modulation dysfunction as follows:
> * Hyperreponsivity, hyporesponsivity or lability in response to sensory stimuli.
> * Unusual patterns of sensory seeking and avoidance.
> * Emotional disregulation evidenced by anxiety, depression, hostility and lability.
> * Attention difficulties including distractibility, disorganization, impulsivity and hyperactivity.
> * Difficulties in functional performance include disruptions in dressing routines, play, mealtime, bath time and social interaction.
> * Poor social participation, insufficient self-regulation and poor self-esteem.

Programming With Modulated Music

An ever-increasing range of CDs is becoming available in the categorization termed modulated music. What appears to be created with the use of modulated music is an 'exercising' effect of the muscles in the middle ear. Flexibility of these muscles is necessary to transmit sensory information to primary sensory processing centers that support sensory modulation, vestibular postural organization and integration and social/cognitive function (see Chapter 2). Biomechanically, it is the function of the middle ear muscles to contract or focus on sounds and relax to monitor the ambient environment. This process should be automatic; however, in many individuals with listening challenges, it seems that the process is not occurring as expected.

Therefore, it is recommended that the vast majority of clients begin a Therapeutic Listening program using modulated music in order to ensure that the middle ear is biomechanically functioning as it should. For some clients with few clinical markers of difficulties with basic modulation and integration, a two week period using modulated music (2x/day, 30 minutes each session) may be sufficient preparation before moving on to other options for a Therapeutic Listening program. For individuals whose primary issues are in sensory modulation and integration, the modulated series of CDs may need to be in place for longer periods of time. An extended listening program may last as long as 10-12 weeks. The greater the difficulty establishing and regulating a functional range of arousal (sleep/wake cycles; bowel/bladder control; hunger/thirst patterns) and grading responses to sensory input, the more extended the Therapeutic Listening program in modulated music. What is critical on an extended program is that the individual listen to the same CD no longer than 3 weeks before a change in the music is made. The change in the music will still be within the modulated music range, but a different CD is needed. This is to ensure that habituation and routinization do not occur.

Clinical Note:
A school age child with mild to moderate sensory defensiveness who has very specific likes and dislikes about clothing and tactile preferences and also has a history of ear infections, yet functions fine in school, may be on a modulated music program for 6-8 weeks.

In contrast, a preschooler who has a very restricted range of foods, doesn't sleep through the night and shows severe sensory defensiveness may be on a modulated music program for up to 10-12 weeks. In addition, when this child moves into SAMONAS, they may still need at least 30 minutes a day of modulated music.

Modulated CDs

- ◆ Alternating high pass/low pass filter.
- ◆ Listening time of 2 X 30 minutes per day (2X 20 minutes/day *Baroque & Mozart String Quartets*).
- ◆ For use only over headphones (a minimum of 3 hours between listening time).
- ◆ Appropriate for individuals with:
  - ◆ a history of chronic middle ear infection or chronic fluid in the middle ear.
  - ◆ sensory modulation disorders (disturbances in sleep/wake cycles, hunger/thirst patterns, bowel/bladder control and other homeostatic functions).
  - ◆ sensory defensiveness.
  - ◆ a history of difficulty grading responses to sensation.
  - ◆ grading functional range of arousal states.
  - ◆ vestibular-auditory-visual integration dysfunction including: postural activation, antigravity responses, midline orientation, postural alignment, coordinating eye, ear and head movement for orientation and localization, visual & auditory figure-ground discrimination.
  - ◆ individuals lacking the biological foundations for social engagement, i.e. facial expression, vocalization, eye contact, etc.
  - ◆ as preparation for other listening programs.

CD Descriptions

EASe Disc 1 and 2

These discs contain 60 minutes of generic synthesized music that has been modulated. No natural instruments have been used. The music has a simple melodic structure. Because the instruments used are electronic, there is little depth or spaciousness to the recordings and there is also little tonal color. Therapeutically, these CDs are equivalent; the numbers do not suggest a hierarchy or progression.

EASe 1 and 2 are an appropriate initial choice in many Therapeutic Listening programs due to the high contrast between auditory foreground and background (higher and lower frequencies) provided by the modulation of the music. The music is suitable for younger listeners and may not hold the attention of many older (7 years of age or older) listeners. EASe 1 or 2 is often an appropriate starting place for individuals with sensory modulation difficulties including hypersensitivity to sound, movement and/or touch or defensive responses to sensory input in general. EASe 1 or 2 is also often the most appropriate starting place for the child with many disruptions in homeostatic functions (i.e. sleep/wake cycles, appetite cycles, bowel/bladder control).

There will undoubtedly be more modulated CDs produced in the coming years. This list reflects what is currently available.

Additionally, the modulation present on *EASe* Disc 1 and 2 appears to create an exercising effect on the muscles of the middle ear, helping to increase the flexibility of the middle ear mechanism. The middle ear plays a critical role in modulating the monitoring vs. focusing aspect of listening. Therefore, *EASe* Disc 1 or 2 is often especially useful for individuals with histories of chronic ear infections, chronic fluid in the middle ear or chronic wax buildup.

EASe Disc 3

This disc also contains 60 minutes of synthesized music that has been modulated. However, many tracks include acoustic instruments (piano and guitar). A further feature is the presence of dolphin and ocean sounds blended with the music. The natural instruments and the presence of nature sounds expands the spatial qualities of the CD.

EASe 3 is far less structured and rhythmically defined than the music of *EASe* 1 or 2. This can make it more challenging for the listener with sensory modulation difficulties who typically seeks more structure and predictability to attain higher levels of organization and integration.

Selection of *EASe* 3 is typically as much personal preference as therapeutic differentiation and may be beneficial for children with modulation difficulties who also seek novelty and whose therapy program would be enhanced by exploring ranges of unpredictability and flexibility. Others have found this CD useful for beginning a Therapeutic Listening program with the child who seems shut down or disconnected. Additionally, dolphin sounds have been likened to the developing child's experience of the mother's voice in utero. This CD might then be beneficial for use with children who have had separation issues at or around the time of birth.

EASe Disc 4

Disc *EASe* 4 contains music that is similar to the music of *EASe* 3. There are a variety of nature sounds present on this CD, again expanding the spatial qualities of the CD.

EASe 4 might be an appropriate starting place for the child who is not focused or connected outwardly and who has poor spatial awareness. It is important to bear in mind that the space captured on *EASe* 4 is not as defined or clear as the space captured on any SAMONAS recording. Use of *EASe* 4 is an appropriate beginning program for the individual with poor spatial organization.

Baroque for Modulation

Baroque for Modulation—Modified is a live recording of a chamber orchestra. The musical selections are both lively and resonant, encouraging movement, postural organization and connection to one's own body. Inherent in the music of the Baroque period is an emphasis on contrast. The musical selections on this CD dynamically contrast tempos, volumes and instrumentation. Contrast between extremes with subsequent ability to maintain organization across a full spectrum is the essence of modulation which therapists seek for their clients.

The chamber orchestra plays compositions from Vivaldi, Quantz and Rameau in the Baroque style that is characterized by orderly, predictable rhythms and harmonic structure. The musical form can alternate between a fast tempo (which captures attention) to a slower tempo which has an impact on physiology (heart rate, respiration, suck/swallow/breathe synchrony, etc.) and can calm and focus attention.

This CD is also rich in overtones without sacrificing a definitive bass line. The lower frequencies provide grounding and organization. The overtones invite attention and engagement outward. For these reasons, this CD may be appropriate for use in the early stages of a Therapeutic Listening program. For some, it may precede use of *EASe* Disc 1 or 2. It is a suitable choice when a client is on an extended Therapeutic Listening program using modulated music (so that a variety of modulated CDs are needed). It may also be beneficial when a client has more subtle modulation issues and may have a difficult time activating his/ her body for successful and sustained interaction with the environment (i.e. the 'low engine' child).

This CD is available in a version that has not been modulated. The modulated version is referred to as *Baroque for Modulation - Modified*. The non-modified speaker version (see Fig. 3-2) may be suitable for use over speakers during meals and transition times as a therapeutic support along with activities that address refinement of midline orientation and the organization of graded postural and respiratory responses. Due to the intensity of the music, listening times are 2 X 20 minutes.

Mozart for Modulation

The pieces for this CD were chosen for the qualities inherent in the music and instrumentation. For example, the Concerto for Two Pianos in E♭ Major promotes directional listening as the pianos play, one and then the other, from different places in space. In all these pieces, the piano provides tones that resonate with and support organized body movement while the flute invites the attention out toward the environment. These qualities support active engagement, blending the internal and external worlds of the listener. The modulation of this CD is similar to that used on the *EASe* discs; however, the instrumentation of the music is more complex.

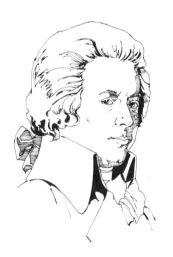

The natural and more complex instrumentation of the music makes this CD an appropriate choice for the older child or adult with sensory modulation difficulties, and it can be suitable for younger children as well. Many times, younger children seem to make a leap in language skills following use of this CD. The inherent dialogue of the musical selections may enhance social skills such as turn taking. The repetition of musical themes with slight variation upon these themes sustains attention and establishes patterns for organization of motor skills and behavior.

This CD is also available in a version that has not been modulated. The modulated version is referred to as *Mozart for Modulation - Modified*. The unmodulated version may be suitable for use over speakers during meals, handwriting groups, transition times, etc. (see Fig. 3-2, p. 3-10).

Mozart String Quartets—Modified I & II

This CD features three Mozart string quartets (two violins, a viola and a cello). In these selections Mozart expanded the quartet model giving all instruments a voice, creating an added complexity. The strings provide a rich overtone structure. The overtone quality of the strings is most similar to the human voice providing a powerful form of emotional expression within the music.

Each piece is composed of four movements and there is a wide variety of emotional and musical expressions, from gay to melancholy, from passionate to technical, from dance movements to slow movements, as well as simple melodies and complex contrapuntal compositions. Contrapuntal compositions weave multiple melodies played by different instruments, into a coherent whole. This increases the complexity of the music. The use of arrhythmic phrases in a rhythmic structure balances novelty and predictably. A wide range of emotional expression along with variety amongst the movements and the balance between novelty and predictability make this music an excellent choice when treatment goals are refinement of self-regulation, language and academic abilities.

This CD is often used toward the end of a modulated listening program as a transition to the use of SAMONAS. The modified version may be particularly intense for some and an initial listening period *may start at 20 minutes.* Not all individuals tolerate the intensity of the strings well, so this CD may not be suitable for all listeners. (see Fig. 3-2, p. 3-10 non-modified version.)

Part of Mozart's genius is the unique impact that his music has on the listener. Each listener may resonate with different emotions expressed in the music. Since Mozart touches on many emotions but does not dwell on them, one might experience sadness but be easily moved to a state of hopefulness. His music tends to reveal more and more with repeated listening. Thus the novelty may last for some time.

Rhythm and Rhyme—Modified
Rhythm and Rhyme is a playful composition of familiar kids' songs that are sung to the accompaniment of piano, guitar and flute. Instrumental improvisation adds an element of novelty. The combination seems to be the right mix of familiarity and novelty to both capture and sustain attention. The instruments and voice are introduced one at a time to gradually increase the complexity and layering of simple melodies. Rhythm is the first element of music to which the infant and younger child responds. The strong rhythms on this CD facilitate the integration of sound with body movement. Rhythmic body movement underlies the body's ability to physically express the motor aspects of communication signals and language. The familiar melodies and rhymes encourage vocalization, singing along and playing with the sounds of the language. This CD may be a good first choice for the preschool child, especially if the introduction of headphones is an issue (see Fig. 3-2, p. 3-10 for non-modulated version).

Kidz Jamz: Grape—Modified (Strawberry & Raspberry, also)
This is a series of instrumental recordings of familiar children's songs. Rhythm is highlighted by a wide variety of drums and other imaginative percussion instruments. Multiple improvisations balanced by the predictability of familiar melodies lends an element of surprise and playfulness to these CDs. Due to the large influence of the rhythms, this is a great starting place for the child with postural organization, sensory modulation and attention difficulties. It has many of the same elements as *Rhythm & Rhyme* and can be used in the same manner.

SAMONAS
and Spectral Activation

Therapeutic Listening incorporates entry-level SAMONAS CDs with Modulated Music into a Sensory Integrative treatment approach. It is important to note that not all professionals who use SAMONAS follow this frame of reference.

SAMONAS sound therapy is a non-generic listening tool that was created by Ingo Steinbach and produced with the utmost quality by Lamdoma. The SAMONAS system can be integrated into a variety of professional practice arenas as an adjunct to other methodology. Spectral Activation is the essential element of the SAMONAS system. Within the system, there are a number of different intensities of Spectral Activation. Less activated CDs up to and including **level one** may be used after participation in an entry level seminar. To be fully trained in SAMONAS, using more intensive spectral activation and sophisticated equipment, one must participate in a five day core training followed by a year of practical experience and written documentation that includes three clearly documented case studies.

All of the recordings in SAMONAS have undergone a special process that maintains the integrity of the harmonic structure through every step of the recording process. This natural form of spectral activation maintains the portion of the sound spectrum that triggers and maintains the listener's attention. This process also maintains the clarity in the portion of the sound spectrum that allows the listener to discriminate between sounds and aids in determining the direction, distance and relative importance of sounds. This higher part carries the finer affective and expressive meaning in the music.

> *All genuine natural sounds have an individual wave form/shape, like a fingerprint. Changes of volume and intensity will alter this fingerprint slightly, without disturbing its identity. The human ability to discriminate sounds is triggered by this individual signature of any natural sound. If we are able to discriminate between the voices of our friends at a party, or to distinguish the teacher's voice from the background noise of the classroom, our auditory system is operating on the variation of the signatures of these acoustic fingerprints.*
>
> *The process of spectral activation intensifies the differences between the tiny variations of sound signatures mirroring their intensity and dynamic range. Spectral activation is like cleaning up a sound and giving it an additional polish to make it easier for the auditory system to identify and discriminate.*
>
> *Steinbach: www.samonas.com*

As discussed above, all the recordings invite spatial listening by preserving and capturing the finer aspects of the recording space. The higher levels of 'entry level SAMONAS' recordings (SE and ST) have undergone a special process that intensifies the spectral activation. Spectral activation enlarges or exaggerates the natural shape of the sound that is created by each sound's individual harmonic pattern. For entry level SAMONAS the increase in volume of spectral harmonics is no more than 4 dB (Steinbach, 2000). The absolute amount of high frequency content of a natural sound is much less when compared with lower frequency content. The entire structure of the ear is adapted to this phenomenon and works to increase the perception of higher frequencies over lower by both its physical structure and in its neurological response.

The ability to discriminate one sound over another is reliant on the ability to pick up the subtle changes or fluctuations in the upper frequency range of any given sound pattern. These differences in sound patterns let us identify one sound over another even when each sound is at the same pitch or frequency, i.e. one voice over another or one instrument over another even when they both sing or play the same note. When passages of music are spectrally activated, it means that the harmonics have been emphasized. Spectral activation acts as a tool for emphasizing the subtle patterns in the natural structure of sounds. This process increases the intensity of the recording as well as highlighting the details in sound.

Programming with SAMONAS

The CDs in the SAMONAS range are necessary for refinement of listening skills and further refining temporal spatial organization, postural organization, higher level attention, auditory selectivity, tonal discrimination, refinement of auditory figure ground and discrimination of the finer aspects of direction and distance of the sound source. The addition of the spatial aspects of listening appears to translate to more accurate perception of space and time across all sensory systems. Spectral activation is used as a tool when more intensity of information is needed to trigger both attention and aid in discrimination. The intensification of contrast in the subtle differences in the upper frequencies highlights and directs attention to the details that are inherent in the harmonic range. It makes sense to use SAMONAS CDs once the ear has been set up by the CDs used in the modulated range. Once the ear has been trained to contract to focus on sounds and relax to monitor the ambient environment, SAMONAS is used to refine the focus and provide more detailed perception of both the temporal and spatial aspects of listening.

Spectral Activation: In a musical passage where the dynamics of the music naturally increase to mark importance or significance and trigger attention, the natural shape of the harmonic structure has been exaggerated by increasing the volume of some harmonics and decreasing the volume of others. This change in the individual volume distribution increases the contrast.

There are several levels of activation available in the SAMONAS range. All recordings were created with the SONAS (Sounds of Optimal Natural Structure) system (see CQ description below). This is not a hierarchy. It is important to match the level of activation with the needs of the individual.

* CQ (*Classic Quality*, SONAS) CDs are naturally spectrally activated. They are selections of classical music recorded to capture and highlight the natural harmonic structure of each instrument by careful placement of microphones. Through this arrangement, the qualities of the space within which the recording occurs are preserved along with the finer frequency content of the harmonic range. Steinbach takes great care in musical selection, instrumentation and quality of the performance. The classic quality recordings (CQ) have not been specifically configured for headphones and may be used over speakers as well as on headphones.

* HS (*Healing Sounds*) CDs are Classic Quality recordings on which frequencies below 300 Hz have been dampened. This makes them appropriate for headphone use only. Both the CQ and HS versions are appropriate for individuals who have a history of strong sensory sensitivities or reactivity particularly to sound (who have already used a modulated CD as a part of a listening program).

* SE and ST SAMONAS recordings undergo a process that intensifies the natural "spectral activation." This process does not disrupt the quality to the overall sound of the music. Additionally, some selections on ST SAMONAS CDs are known as "high extension" passages. These are brief passages of music where only the high harmonics remain; the overall volume of these passages of music will seem quite soft and the ears will have to "reach" for the sound. The SAMONAS *Entry* (SE) and *Sound Therapy* (ST) level of CDs are used for individuals who seem to need a lot more information and/or intensity to be able to demonstrate improvements in functional skill and organization. These CDs are very appropriate for the individual who needs more intensity to capture and maintain attention. Spectral Activation is appropriate when an individual has difficulty discriminating more detailed aspects of sounds such as detecting tonal differences, phonemic awareness, as well as the discriminating the temporal and spatial aspects of sounds and language. SE may be more appropriate for the younger child who needs the details and sound structure emphasized. ST is often necessary for the school age child who needs more intensity and more information.

Since these CDs are more intensive in terms of details and finer discrimination than the modulated CDs, the listening times are much shorter. An initial listening time is 5 minutes, with incremental increases by one minute every fourth day as long as change continues in an organized progression and disorganization does not occur. Some children who are very sensitive may listen less than 5 minutes. *There is no set goal of attaining a certain listening time*. Most children listen somewhere between 5 and 15 minutes daily with a very positive result.

Right ear weighting

In addition, most of the SE and ST CDs have been weighted (slightly more volume) to the right ear. The right ear has more connections with the left hemisphere which is the dominant hemisphere for language in 98% of the population. Even a large percentage of left-handed individuals are left hemisphere dominant for language (Madaule, 1997).

The CQ and HS CDs are not weighted. The SEs have a very slight weighting of 1-2 dB to the right. The STs are weighted 2-3 dB's to the right with the exception of two CDs: the *Romantic* has no weighting due to its primary purpose in inducing affect and expression which is more of a feature of the right hemisphere. The other exception is the ST version of *Carulli* that is strongly weighted to the right by 6-8 dB. This is meant to facilitate the left hemisphere not only in language functions, but to stimulate temporal and sequential processing that is associated with left hemisphere functions.

Programming with SAMONAS

♦ Appropriate for individuals who have therapeutic needs in the areas of temporal-spatial organization (vestibular, auditory, visual and sensorimotor), higher level postural organization and praxis, higher level attention, auditory selectivity and discrimination.

♦ CQ - naturally spectrally activated; recorded according to Ingo Steinbach's meticulous specifications.

♦ CQ - may be used over speakers which alters the impact of listening.

♦ CQ - may be used as background music for a handwriting group, transitions within a classroom, etc.

♦ CQ and HS - appropriate for individuals who have a history of sensitivity or reactivity to sensation, particularly sound (who may have already used a modulated CD as part of a listening program).

♦ HS - frequencies below 300 Hz have been dampened.

♦ SE (SAMONAS Entry) - spectrally activated to a lesser degree than ST (Sound Therapy - SAMONAS Level 1).

♦ HS, SE and ST - meant only for headphones.

♦ Initial listening time of 5 minutes 1x per day, adding 1 minute every 4th day.

♦ SE and ST - used for individuals who seem to need a lot of information or intensity in order to demonstrate improvements in functional skill and organization.

All SAMONAS recordings may have an impact on emotionality. Listening time and disc choices are critical to outcomes.

SAMONAS - CD Descriptions

01 - Classic - Flute, Harp and Cello
(Available in CQ, HS, SE, ST versions)

This CD contains music of flute, harp and cello from the Classic Period of music history. The melodies are clear, clean and simple. This simplicity is maintained for the duration of the CD and is an important consideration for some listeners for whom musical complexity might prove overbearing.

Within the recording, the cello provides grounding and connection to body; the harp plays a background rhythm and marks time; the flute relates to human voice and breath and creates the melodic line that draws postural and perceptual attention outward and invites engagement. The rhythms of the CD as well as the use of flute (a breath instrument) seem to correlate well with the basic suck/swallow/breathe synchrony. Use of this CD often promotes coordination of this synchrony. In general, it is also been found helpful in deepening respiration for relaxation and for promoting more refined oral motor skill.

There will undoubtedly be more SAMONAS CDs produced in the coming years. This list reflects what is currently available.

02 - Romantic - Flute, Harp and Cello
(Available in CQ, HS, SE, ST versions)

The music of flute, harp and cello on this CD is from the Romantic Period of music history and, as the name suggests, is quite emotionally evocative. The melodies are flowing and poignant. Though relatively 'easy' in structure, the rhythms are not as repetitive or clearly defined as on 01 - *Classic*. Also, unlike 01 - *Classic*, the musical selections gain complexity as the CD progresses. Additionally, the richness of the harmonic structure increases the relative complexity of this CD.

The emotional tone of this CD is its prevailing feature. The cello provides a point of attachment to the physical while the flute and harp play on emotion, facilitating connection to self and others in the present moment.

These qualities make this CD uniquely suited for bringing forth emotion and with emotion, greater physical and verbal expressiveness. This CD, then, may be an appropriate choice for individuals with difficulty expressing emotion (both verbally and non-verbally) or linking emotion to action and interaction. It may be a less desirable choice for those individuals with a tendency toward emotional lability or mood disregulation.

03 - Carulli
(Available in CQ, HS, SE, ST versions)

The music of the composer *Carulli* is very rhythmical and structured. There is a high degree of predictability to the musical pattern. The rhythm is almost obligatory in nature. It marks time in a manner from which it is difficult to deviate. The instrumentation of piano and guitar is rich in overtone structure which promotes attention, yet the lower register of both the piano and guitar strongly organizes the body through time. Rhythm and timing are the chief features of this CD.

This CD is an appropriate selection for the individual who does not seem connected to his/her body and has difficulty with midline organization and integration between upper and lower extremities or right and left sides of the body. Changes in postural activation and organization, praxis, initiation, sequencing and timing are often observed following use of *Carulli* in a Therapeutic Listening program. This CD is also appropriate for those with difficulty with temporal organization, and changes in handwriting and visual motor-integration are not uncommon following use of this CD in a Therapeutic Listening program. Additionally, due to its very insistent rhythmical qualities, this CD is also appropriate for use with those individuals who seem to lack internal rhythm.

04 - Live in Catalunya - Music of Rossini, Grieg & Tchaikovsky (referred to as "Chamber") (Available in CQ, HS, ST versions)

The music of this CD is more musically complex than that of *Carulli*; however, rhythmicity and structure are still clearly defined. The stringed instrumentation of the chamber orchestra represents a full range of frequencies low to high. This layering and complexity of sounds as well as the cathedral in which the recording occurred lend a rich spatial quality that is a hallmark of this CD. The spaciousness captured here is a defined or bounded space as opposed to the environmental space captured on ST 110 *Sounds of Nature*.

Wide variation of musical styles is represented by the three composers whose selections are used on this CD. Rossini, who began composing at an early age, is relatively more playful and light-spirited in nature. Grieg's music has a heavy, more somber quality to it. Tchaikovsky's musical arrangements are quite complex.

The variations in the musical compositions and the 'full container of sound' with its preservation of the inherent spatial essence of the moment of recording make this CD an appropriate choice for individuals with subtle sensory modulation difficulties, especially when the modulation difficulties are coupled with challenges in postural organization, modulation of respiration, learning, language and temporal-spatial organization. Often this CD is an appropriate choice for a more musically sophisticated child or for an adult for whom *Carulli* may not sustain interest and attention. Because the music of this CD is less patterned and repetitive than that of *Carulli*, it can be an appropriate selection for the individual who gets stuck in repetition to the exclusion of flexibility and spontaneity.

05 - Cadaques Night - Music of Three Guitars
(Available in CQ, HS, SE versions)

The hallmark of this CD is the joyfulness that clearly emanates from the musicians. Recorded improvisationally, this element adds to the joyful, playful spirit of the music. The spatial essence of the recording is again cleanly preserved; however, the space is small, well-defined and uncluttered.

The three guitars create less novelty in harmonic structure than a variety of instruments played together might. One guitar typically provides a background rhythm while another guitar plays the melody. The resonance of the guitars is in itself physically connecting and organizing.

A range of musical compositions is also represented on the CD. Classical, jazz and flamenco compositions are all present. The range of styles promotes attentiveness. The rhythmical complexity of this CD tends to capture and sustain attention; however, on most selections the rhythm is defined enough to provide clarity and order.

08 - Music of Mozart and Contemporaries II
(Available in CQ, HS, SE versions)

Symmetry is an element essential to Mozart's style. His music is rhythmically balanced and often has an almost conversational nature. Frequently, there is a call and response in the composition of the music; one instrument plays the melody and another echoes it back with a slight variation. Additionally, Mozart's creations contain a regularity of tempo that is very organizing, especially for the more refined levels of organization needed for cognitive and academic tasks.

On this particular Mozart recording, Steinbach selected a wooden flute rather than a silver flute. The tone of the wooden flute is not as 'bright' or sharp as that of the silver flute. This makes the frequency range and tonal color of the wooden flute closely related to human voice.

This CD is an appropriate selection when refinement of pragmatic and conversational language and social skills are goals. Additionally, this CD may be useful in promoting organization around academics.

10 - Sounds of Nature
(Available in ST version)

There is no music at all on this CD, only the sounds of birds, wind and water. There are no predictable patterns present, and this may be an important consideration for some individuals. The most salient feature of this CD is again the space within which it was recorded. However, space is now environmental space, an open, expansive space rather than a space bounded by walls.

There are only three tracks on this CD. The first is birds in the morning, the second is birds in the evening and the third follows the journey of a stream from the mountains down in to a valley. Each track has a distinctly different mood and can be matched to the current needs of the client.

This CD is extremely helpful for individuals who lack a solid perceptual understanding and awareness of three-dimensional space. It is often useful for the individual termed 'defensive' but whose defensive characteristics stem from poor spatial awareness rather than heightened reactivity to sensation. These individuals most often present a clinical picture of being sensitive or 'defensive' to lower frequency sounds (vacuum cleaner, public toilets, hair dryer, thunder, fireworks, chain saw, lawn mower, etc.) that give little spatial information. This CD may be less useful for individuals with clear sensitivities to higher pitched sounds as the birds are quite sharp and distinct.

21 - Nocturne
(Available in CQ, HS versions)

The music on *Nocturne* is played by flute and guitar. The initial melodies are simple and even familiar; however, the music gains complexity as the CD progresses. The warmth of the lower range of the guitar provides a clear tempo around which body movements can be organized. The higher register of the flute helps capture attention.

This CD may be an appropriate selection in a Therapeutic Listening program for younger children as the grounding and centering effects of the guitar may be helpful in promoting body awareness and postural organization. With the body centered by the guitar, the flute then invites attention outward for engagement and interaction.

22 - Cantabile
(Available in CQ, HS, versions)

The music on *Cantabile* is played by flute and harp. Like *Nocturne*, the initial melodies are simple and become more complex as the CD progresses. The CD ranges from somber to bright in mood, dependent upon each individual musical selection. The harp provides structure while the flute carries the melody.

This CD lightly evokes emotion and may be useful for the more sensitive individual for whom *02 Romantic* is too intense.

23 - Lascia Ch'io Pianga
(Available in CQ, HS versions)

This recording is of an operatic mezzo-soprano. Human voice is the primary instrument and thus has great potential for connection and attachment. The vocalist is accompanied only by the simple clear strains of the guitar which provides warmth and a background rhythm to the recording. This CD is highly emotionally evocative because of the draw to human connection and attachment.

Therapeutically, this CD can be used in much the same manner and for the same considerations as *02 Romantic*.

ASSESSMENT

Assessment procedures for selecting and implementing a Therapeutic Listening program are no different than the assessment procedures one might normally use. For example: an occupational therapist will evaluate motor skills, perception, sensory processing and functional, daily life skills; a speech pathologist will assess oral motor skills and all levels of communication; a teacher will measure a child's academic progress. All disciplines will likely use a variety of assessment tools including standardized evaluations, observation of the child in functional tasks, an interview with the child, the child's family and other relevant caregivers and professionals. Information collected from observation as well as from interview is equally as valuable and pertinent as information garnered from standardized procedures. It is the information gained in these informal ways that may provide the most accurate picture of the child's performance over time rather than during one window of opportunity.

Before a child begins a Therapeutic Listening program it is critical that the therapist has current audiological information to rule out hearing loss and to evaluate the middle ear for the presence of fluid. Information gathered from an audiological assessment measures the sensation or detection of sound, or the ability to identify the presence of sound. An audiological assessment may also document auditory thresholds (how sensitive one can hear throughout the frequency range) and tolerance levels. Tolerance levels assesses one's comfort with and ability tolerate decibel or volume levels throughout the frequency range.

Auditory Defensiveness

Auditory defensiveness has been defined by the Wilbargers (1991, p. 4) as, "oversensitivity to certain sounds and may involve irritable or fearful responses to noises like vacuum cleaners, motors, fire alarms, etc."

Because of the variability of symptoms, when a sensory history reveals auditory defensiveness it is important to gain more information regarding the qualities of the sounds to which the child is reacting. Individual differences in reactivity to sound patterns will provide valuable information for treatment planning.

Apparent overreactivity to low frequency sounds

Overreactivity is commonly interpreted as a sensitivity to sound. In the case of low frequency sounds it is actually due to an inability to differentiate spatial cues present in this frequency range (below 300-500 Hz). Since sounds in this range are multi-directional and do not contain much spatial information, they may overwhelm the individual, causing fearful, defensive, flight, fright reactions. The vacuum cleaner, the lawn mower and public toilets are examples of the sounds that these individuals may not be able to localize. They may need to maintain visual contact with the source of the sound to feel comfortable (Figs. 3-3).

Individuals may also respond defensively to sounds within other frequency ranges as irritable or threatening, such as vocal patterns or very high pitched sounds. Again it is helpful to try to get an impression regarding which frequency range and at what intensity level these sounds occur (Figs. 3-4 through 3-8).

Loud sounds in the range from 90 dB up to 120 dB are typically uncomfortable. Individuals who experience discomfort in loud situations and can continue to function are displaying a normal response. However, individuals with defensiveness may experience exaggerated responses and a disruption in functional skill to sounds in this volume range as well as to sounds at much quieter levels. Some individuals may exhibit irritable and fearful responses to very quiet sounds in the low frequency range, such as air vents or motor sounds in the distance. This is often the case with those who are very tactually defensive. These sounds are perceived by the body through the tactile and vibratory receptors (Fig. 3-6).

Using the charts in Figs. 3-3 through 3-8 as a guide, make an attempt to analyze sound patterns according to the frequencies and decibel levels that cause difficulties for the individual.

The inability to filter out the irrelevant sounds in complex acoustic environments may also lead to difficulties. These difficulties may present as distractibility and inattentiveness. They can occur in response to any frequency range at any intensity (volume) level. These difficulties will be evident in the results from subtests of the SCAN and the Test of Auditory Discrimination coupled with functional information gathered from a sensory history (p. 3-30).

As in other forms of defensiveness and/or other sensory processing dysfunction, specific sound patterns and certain auditory environments can create changeable levels of distress and anxiety. Distress to sounds over periods of time may lead to unresponsiveness due to auditory overload or shut down.

Since listening is a whole body function it is important to assess not only functional and sensory processing skills in the auditory domain but all levels of function, especially those areas impacted heavily by sensations that are processed through the vestibular system (see p. 3-42 for treatment suggestions).

Following assessment, determination of goals for treatment occurs. These goals are based upon what is significant for the child across functional environments. The family's goals for the child are always regarded, even if they must be broken down incrementally or into more fundamental steps. Treatment planning for the child then develops based upon assessment results and stated goals.

Assessments Chart

Assessment	Age Range	Description
The Sensory Profile Dunn 1998	Appropriate for 3-10 years	Caregivers complete a 125-item questionnaire reporting the frequency with which their child responds to various sensory experiences. It can be used to determine how well children ages 3 to 10 process sensory information in everyday situations. It profiles the sensory systems' effects on functional performance. The items are grouped into three major sections: sensory processing, modulation and behavioral and emotional responses.
Autism Treatment Evaluation Checklist (ATEC) Rimland and Edelson 1999	No age recommended	This form is intended to measure the effects of treatment across the domains of Speech/Language/Communication; Sociability; Sensory/Cognitive Awareness; Health/Physical/Behavioral. Free scoring is available on the internet at www.autism.com/ari.
Peabody Developmental Motor Scales Folio & Fewell 1983	Appropriate for birth to 83 months.	Measures gross and fine motor development on a broad scale. There is a revised edition available, but the authors prefer the older version for measuring discreet changes.
Developmental Test of Visual Motor Integration Beery and Buktenica 1997	Appropriate for age 2-15	Measures visual perceptual, motor control and visual motor integration for design copying items.
Minnesota Handwriting Assessment Reisman, 1999	Appropriate for first and second graders	Rates the five qualitative aspects of legibility, form, alignment, size and spacing of both manuscript and D'Nealian handwriting.
Goodenough-Harris Draw a Person Harris 1963	Standardizes scores from age 3-15.	Measures conceptual maturity and has been shown to correlate with intellectual development. It may be used to gain an initial impression of a young child's general ability level.
Sensorimotor Performance Analysis (SPA) Richter & Montgomery, 1989	Ages 4 to adult	Criterion referenced assessment designed to provide a qualitative record of individual performance on gross and fine motor tasks. An excellent measure for assessing the components of movement patterns and postural control.

The following tests deal with general auditory processing and are not meant for diagnostic purposes. They may help to validate behavioral and functional difficulties related to more complex auditory environments. They also provide some pre/post data to further validate functional improvements following intervention. Each therapy setting will dictate the most appropriate professional background for administering the following assessments.

SCAN-C The Test For Auditory Processing Disorders in Children	Ages 3 to 11 years	The SCAN is a screening test for auditory processing disorders. It can be used to assess auditory development and screen for level of efficiency in auditory processing skills. The SCAN is used in an academic setting for children with poor listening skills and or difficulty learning through the auditory channel. The SCAN may also be useful in obtaining information about how an individual processes auditory stimuli.
SCAN-A: A test for Auditory Processing Disorders in Adolescents and Adults Keith, 2000	Ages 12 to Adult	
The Test of Auditory Perceptual Skills (TAPS) Gardener, 1985	Ages 4 to 11	The TAPS was designed to aid in assessing the specific areas of language based auditory skills that will impact the child's ability to learn to read and spell. It includes six language based auditory skills: auditory number memory, auditory sentence memory, auditory word memory, auditory interpretation of directions, auditory word discrimination and thinking and reasoning.
Goldman- Fristoe- Woodcock Test Of Auditory Discrimination Goldman, Fristoe, Woodcock. 1970	Ages 4 to adult	The GFW is designed to provide measures of speech sound discrimination with few confounding factors. It provides a measure of auditory processing of speech under an ideal quiet listening condition as well as a comparative measure in the presence of controlled background noise.
Lindamood Auditory Conceptualization Lindamood, 1971	Ages preschool to adult	The Lindamood is a test designed to measure auditory perception and conceptualization of speech sounds. The LAC measures ability to judge auditorily the identity, number and the sequence of sounds in spoken patterns and the ability to conceptualize the points of contrast between sound patterns.

Examples of documentation with assessments (see also Chapter 4)

Malea

Malea's scores on the **Sensory Profile** indicated marked change in the following areas after six weeks of her treatment program: 1) Sensory Sensitivity, Sedentary and Touch Processing factors shifted from a score indicating a definite difference to a score indicating a typical performance. 2) Vestibular Processing and Modulation Related to Body Position and Movement shifted from a score indicating a <u>definite difference</u> to a score indicating <u>typical performance</u>. Malea's mother also reported that she now enjoys playing on the playground equipment, including swings; she is less emotionally reactive throughout her day; transitions more easily and is more socially engaging with those outside her family.

Dylan

Dylan is a 7 year old boy with a diagnosis of autism. He presented with difficulties with modulating arousal level, receptive and expressive language skills, poor articulation and limited eye contact and social skills. On July 5, 2000 Dylan's total score **ATEC** <u>score was 66</u> placing him on the scale in the moderate range of impairment. He began a Therapeutic Listening program with no other therapeutic intervention at that time. On July 30, Dylan's total **ATEC** <u>score was 36</u> which barely place him in the mild range of impairment. Dylan's mother reported calmer, more confident behavior; he was able to listen and follow directions better; he had better eye contact and more creative speech with improved articulation. He was also able to rapidly progress through levels of a computer program called "Earobics" which had been impossible for him prior to listening.

Thomas

This 10 year old was referred for a Therapeutic Listening program due to auditory defensiveness. Loud noises or unexpected noises in an otherwise quiet environment bothered him. This problem was affecting his performance at school and his family's ability to enjoy events such as dining in restaurants. His listening program consisted of *Mozart for Modulation -Modified, EASe 1 and ST 102.* **The Screening Test of Auditory Processing (SCAN)** was administered prior to his listening and again following his program. The results were as follows:

	2/10	4/28
Filtered Words	SS = 11	SS = 16
	63%	98%
Auditory Figure-Ground	SS = 3	SS = 8
	1%	25%

Competing Words	SS = 4	SS = 12
	2%	75%
SCAN Composite	SS = 65	SS = 109
	1%	73%
	AE = 5.7	AE = 11.0

In the span of two months Thomas attained age appropriate performance. Functionally he continued to demonstrate some sensitivity in noisy environments, however his coping strategies in those situations have been more adaptive.

Sara

This 7 year old girl's parents questioned her speech and language skills since approximately 18 months of age. Sara's formalized testing consisted of the **Goldman-Fristoe-Woodcock Test of Auditory Discrimination**, which is designed to provide measures of speech-sound discrimination ability under ideal listening conditions plus a comparative measure of auditory discrimination in the presence of controlled background noise. Sara performed at the first percentile for both the quiet and noise subtest.

A home program of Disc *EASe* for two 30-minute sessions a day was implemented. The testing was repeated after three weeks with significant changes noted. She went from the first percentile to the 70th percentile for the quiet subtest and to the 84th percentile on the noise subtest (p. 4-35).

Jack

Jack is a 5 year old who was referred to occupational therapy for significant developmental delays across all domains (see p. 4-49-4-53). His initial scores on the **Peabody Developmental Motor Scales** at 63 months of age were:

Gross Motor	36 months
Fine Motor	50 months
Age Equivalent	48 months

Draw-A-Person Score: 2 years

Following 10 months (73 months of age) on a Therapeutic Listening program consisting of a series of modulated music and ST 101, his scores reflect considerable improvement:

Gross Motor	67 months
Fine Motor	83 months
Age Equivalent	75 months

Draw-A-Person	7 years

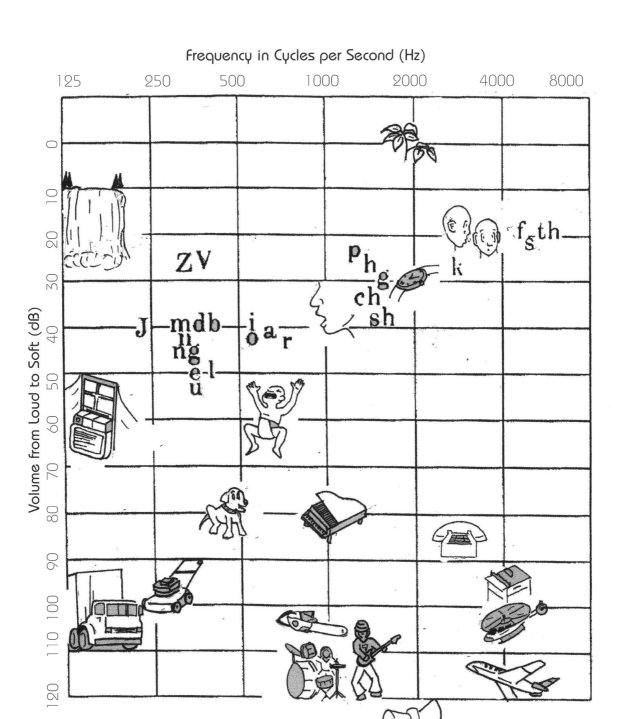

This chart identifies the frequency spectrum of familiar sounds plotted on a standard audiogram (source unknown). This may be useful in determining the characteristics (what frequency-HZ and at what volumes-dB) of sounds that create defensive reactions and negative behavioral responses.

Fig. 3-3

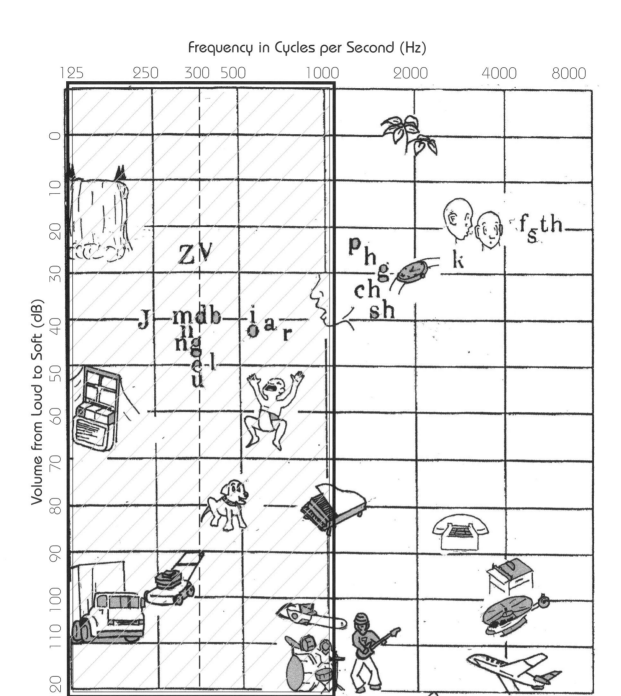

Sounds in the range of 125 - 1000 Hz are related to rhythmic movement and gross motor skill. Sounds below 300 Hz contain little spatial information. Individuals who do not understand space may find these sounds threatening due to the inability to localize them.

Fig. 3-4

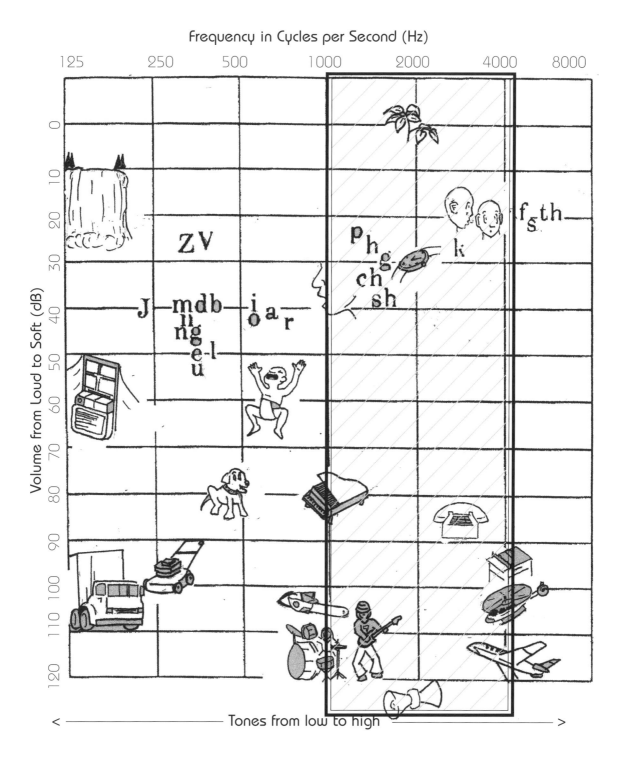

Sounds in the 1000-4000 Hz range contain key elements for recognizing the human voice and speech sounds. Distortions in this range may affect auditory attention to speech and possibly articulation.

Fig. 3-5

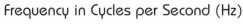

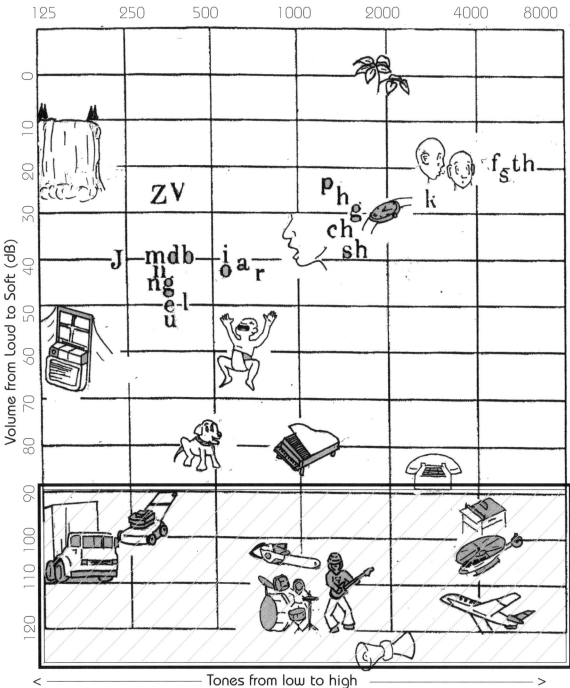

Sound levels between 90-120 dB are reported as uncomfortable. Audiologists and some Speech/Language Pathologists may perform tests at uncomfortable loudness levels. Individuals with difficulties in sensory modulation may also respond to much quieter sounds as uncomfortable.

Fig. 3-6

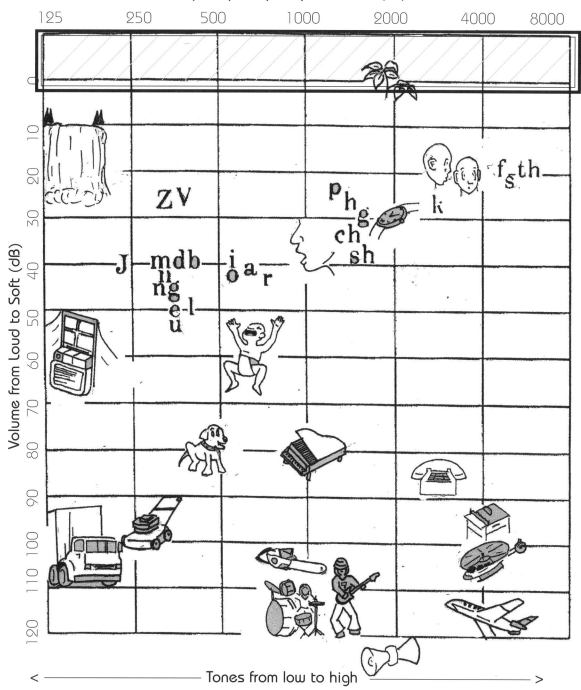

Frequency in Cycles per Second (Hz)

Volume from Loud to Soft (dB)

< ——————————— Tones from low to high ——————————— >

Range of hearing that is above average threshold and may be reported as hyperacusis. This may be picked up on threshold audiogram testing. Some individuals report pain in this range.

Many individuals with hyperacusis will be hypersensitive or become disorganized, uncomfortable or emotionally reactive. These individuals who are very sensitive to sounds may also easily overload and appear to shut down to auditory input in complex acoustic environments.

Fig. 3-7

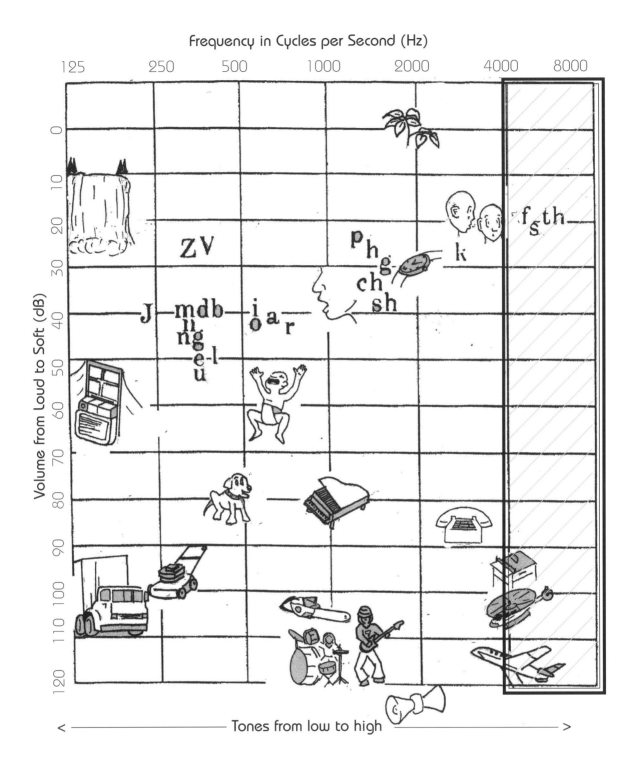

Frequency in Cycles per Second (Hz)

Volume from Loud to Soft (dB)

Tones from low to high

Sounds between 4000-8000 Hz typically trigger our attention and difficulties or distortions in this range may be related to difficulties attending and processing sounds for details.

Fig. 3-8

TREATMENT IMPLEMENTATION

A basic model for implementing treatment from a sensory integration frame of reference has previously been set forth by Oetter, et al (1995). The elements of this treatment model are **frequency, duration, intensity and rhythm.** These elements apply beautifully to the integration of a Therapeutic Listening program into a holistic treatment plan.

Frequency relates to how often an activity is required for an individual to maintain a desired level or state of organization. The frequency of a Therapeutic Listening program varies with the music selected and each individual. When using modulated music, it is unusual to deviate from a listening time of 2x/day, 30 minutes each session, separated by a minimum of 3 hours. However, when SAMONAS is introduced into a Therapeutic Listening program, listening times can vary widely. Most individuals listen 1x per day, for 5-15 minutes. Some individuals may listen longer during their listening session; some individuals may benefit from listening 2x per day. Rarely, a very sensitive individual might listen for less than 5 minutes and still benefit from the music selected.

Duration refers to the length of time that the input is needed. Most listening programs go through a series of evolutions or progressions. (**Remember: changes should be made in the CDs every 2-3 weeks.**) A typical length of time to listen might be 6-12 months. If an individual listens daily for longer than 6 months, it is likely that several breaks from listening occurred during this time frame. It would not be unusual for listening to become part of an ongoing sensory diet. In this circumstance, listening might be ongoing in some fashion for longer than a year. Again, breaks from listening might occur or listening might occur several times per week rather than on a daily basis if this is the situation.

Intensity correlates to the power of the input involved. With respect to a Therapeutic Listening program, intensity is measured in several ways. The way in which the music has been modified is one measure of intensity. Generally speaking, CDs that have been spectrally activated provide more intensity to higher cortical structures than those that are modulated. The instrumentation used on a CD is another gauge of intensity. Electronic instruments produce sounds with simpler wave patterns than do natural instruments, thus they produce sounds that are less intense. While instruments that play in lower frequency ranges of sound (i.e. cello, guitar) are more intense for somatosensory functions they are less intense than those that play in

In this model rhythm refers to the ratio between novelty and repetition.

higher frequency ranges (i.e. flute, violin) for higher levels of attention/engagement and more cortically driven functions. Finally, the musical composition itself will have a relative intensity. Some compositions are significantly more emotional in tone than others. For most listeners, the music of *Carulli* provides order and structure and does not deeply stir the emotions while the music of *Romantic* is very emotionally evocative and poignant.

Finally, **rhythm** must be considered. Obviously, each of the CDs will provide some sort of rhythm. Again, the rhythms of *Carulli* are very ordered and predictable. The rhythmic structure of *Romantic* is more open and fluid. *Sounds of Nature* contains no predictable rhythm. The degree to which rhythm is necessary to promote organization for an individual will vary greatly. If sequencing and timing are issues, a strong rhythmic pulse is helpful. If an individual is very order-bound and flexibility is a goal, then less rhythmic compositions may be beneficial. Additionally, rhythm may refer to the time of day during which listening occurs. Every individual has his/her own diurnal rhythms. Listening at certain times of the day (i.e. upon awakening, after lunch) may promote alertness and organization for some. Listening at other times (i.e. after 5 p.m. or immediately prior to bed time) may create a degree of disorganization for some individuals.

As with designing any plan of intervention, all of these aspects need to be considered when implementing a Therapeutic Listening program. Which factors are most crucial for which individuals will vary. Additionally, changing one factor (i.e. intensity) may necessitate changing another factor (i.e. frequency).

Initial Therapeutic Listening Protocol

Determining an initial Therapeutic Listening program is straightforward. In the broad majority of cases, some form of modulated music is selected first. The length of the program of modulated music will vary considerably based upon the individual's characteristics and behaviors. Modulated music is selected first because it seems to facilitate the desired biomechanical function of the middle ear leading to improvement in subcortical sensory integrative processes.

The length of the modulated music program typically varies from 2-12 weeks. An individual with a history of middle ear infections but little history of sensory modulation difficulties might listen to modulated music for only 2 weeks. An individual with a previous history of mild-to-moderate sensory defensiveness, sensory modulation and vestibular-auditory-visual based dysfunction might listen to modulated music for 6-8 weeks. The individual who has difficulties maintaining basic physiological homeostasis might listen to modulated music for 10-12 weeks.

Any extended listening program using modulated music for longer than 2-3 weeks should be varied in the CDs utilized. Variety in the CDs will facilitate flexibility and help prevent habituation. An individual listening to modulated music for 10-12 weeks may have 4-6 different modulated CDs in his or her listening library.

Adding SAMONAS to a
Therapeutic Listening Program

Following use of modulated music, one of two SAMONAS CDs is most often used next: *Carulli* or *Sounds of Nature*. These two CDs provide the biggest impact on spatial-temporal organization. *Carulli* facilitates temporal organization; *Sounds of Nature* facilitates spatial organization. The order in which the CDs are introduced into a Therapeutic Listening program is determined by which of these two areas is of greatest concern for the individual.

In most cases, individuals will use both of these CDs, one following the other. One might be introduced while the first is still in use, creating a 'blended' listening program. The total time of this blended program is equal to the amount of time on a single CD. Additionally, it is possible (and in many cases likely) that the individual may begin on *Carulli* or *Sounds of Nature* while continuing on one session per day of modulated music.

EASe 1 & 2, Rhythm & Rhyme, Kidz Jamz and *Mozart for Modulation - Modified* are the first selections for improving sensory modulation and vestibular-auditory-visual integration.
EASe 3 & 4 work well for individuals who are more shut down and lack connection and basic engagement.
Baroque & Mozart String Quartets I & II provide more intensity for those needing more input, i.e. low tone, slow to arouse or activate. Recommended times are 20 minutes rather than 30. This has worked well with adults with auditory defensiveness. The *Mozart String Quartets* can be a good transition from an extended modulated music program to SAMONAS.

If the individual exhibits many signs of poor body awareness, poor postural organization, decreased midline orientation and decreased praxis (especially sequencing and timing), *Carulli* is the most appropriate next choice. The level of activation of the *Carulli* CD must be carefully selected to appropriately match the individual's needs.
If the individual exhibits poor spatial awareness, a lack of 'connection' to the environment, or seems especially sensitive to lower frequency, non-directional sounds (vacuum cleaners, thunder, public toilets, blenders, lawn mowers, etc.), then *Sounds of Nature* would be the next logical choice.

Therapeutic Listening
Initial Listening Protocol

Modulated Music
· *EASe, Rhythm & Rhyme, Kidz Jamz, Baroque, Mozart*
· 2-12 weeks based upon degree of modulation issues
· change discs every 2-3 weeks to avoid habituation

Introducing SAMONAS
Carulli
· choose level of activation based upon sensitivity of client
· 3-4 weeks based upon response
· may be blended with modulated music
· use first following modulated music if issues are about:
postural activation; midline organization;
temporal organization;
timing & sequencing elements of praxis

Sounds of Nature
· 3-4 weeks based upon response
· blend modulated music
· use first following modulated music if issues are about:
spatial organization;
sensitivity to lower frequency, non-directional sounds

Concurrent Treatment

Just as professionals will assess the client through their discipline-specific lenses, so then should treatment occur. All other tools in the professional's tool bag should be used to enhance the outcomes of a Therapeutic Listening program. Listening often creates opportunities and hastens the speed at which outcomes are met. However, newly emergent skills must be supported by a solid foundation. A well-planned sensory diet is a critical part of any treatment regimen. Activities that promote postural activation and organization along with graded respiration help to maintain modulation and organization and often 'cement' newly emerging perceptual and motor skills. Skills that emerge must be challenged and used in activities that are meaningful to the individual for if not used functionally, they may not become integrated (Kimball, 1993.)

Posture

The inner ear is not only responsible for listening to the sounds of our environment; the vestibular portion is also responsible for detecting movement both of the environment and of our bodies. The vestibular system is important in defining one's relationship to gravity and also providing the reference point of where one is in space. The vestibular system has diffuse connections to other lower centers in the brain including the reticular formation (regulates arousal, attention, alertness) and the limbic system (emotional tone, basic drives & memory). Because of its bilateral representation, the vestibular system is especially important in helping coordinate the two sides of the body. The vestibular system, through its connections with the cerebellum, also plays a role in mediating postural tone and organizing postural and movement strategies. Postural organization, or postural adaptation refers to the automatic movements that are necessary to orient our bodies and adapt them to changes in the environment. Information from our vestibular structures contributes significantly to our ability to dynamically adjust our posture, allowing for the positioning of the body for the most efficient movements relative to the chosen task.

Many of the children and adults who experience listening difficulties show subtle difficulties with postural organization and use a limited repertoire of movement strategies. Inefficient processing of the sensations of both sound and movement often lead to these difficulties. Clinical observations and assessment often reveal that these individuals lack balanced use of many of the primary movement patterns and early developing antigravity responses to movement.

Ayres (1979) pointed out the importance of development of the antigravity responses and their relationship to the sensory integrative process. She discussed the relationship between the early development of the antigravity responses and their critical significance in sensory registration and the orienting responses needed throughout life. All humans have an innate drive to master gravity, to pull up to the vertical and balance the body relative to the pull of gravity. This is accomplished first on the belly, next on all fours and eventually in the upright position. Once upright is mastered the drive continues to challenge gravity and refine skills in jumping, hopping, climbing, etc. The antigravity responses also allow us to pull upward, direct the face forward and begin to relate to vision and hearing in the horizontal plane. A body that is able to right itself against gravity and make adjustments in accordance with the environment is in a position for alertness, attention and competent interaction with the environment.

Oetter (1986) termed this phenomenon 'postural attention'. Difficulties with postural attention are often secondary to inefficient and unbalanced development of antigravity extension and flexion. The results can be poorly developed and inefficient use of righting, rotation, midline stability and equilibrium - functions that are critical foundations for self organization, attention in toward the body and building gross and fine motor patterns. This in turn hampers perception since these patterns provide the postural basis that enables an individual to receive consistent information about the body and its relationship to the environment in terms of space, place and time.

The increased use of extension without balanced flexion leaves the body open and vulnerable to the whole sensory environment (near and far). This draws attention outward to vigilance and monitoring and reinforces flight, fright and fight motor patterns. This may create difficulty screening out environmental stimuli and reinforce distractibility and hypervigilance, which will in turn impact attention and behavioral organization. Conversely, lack of antigravity extension, or a less alert and upright posture may result in a tendency to be pulled passively into flexion toward the forces of gravity, which make the individual less available (visually, auditorily and tactually). This passive flexion may result in less vigilance along with difficulty orienting and engaging.

Furthermore, poorly organized postural patterns also lead to further inefficiencies in processing sensory information due to inadequate or inaccurate information to and from muscles and tendons. This information provides the reference point for the body in space and helps one make sense of information received from the body and the environment for more sophisticated temporal spatial organization of sensation and movement. The organization of sensation allows orientation to and discrimination of more discrete information from the body and the environment. Any imbalance in the basic components of movement will impact the reception and processing of sensation as well as how organized a response will be to any given sensation.

Clinical experience indicates that individuals on listening programs begin to have a better understanding of the three dimensionality of space. They begin to move their bodies more efficiently in ways that challenge gravity and refine movement and postural organization. This refined sense of gravity, better understanding of their body in space, increased orientation towards midline and more accurate perceptions of the surrounding environmental space appears to facilitate changes in postural organization. Combining activities that encourage and support further postural organization and refinement furthers the process of sensory integration and functional change.

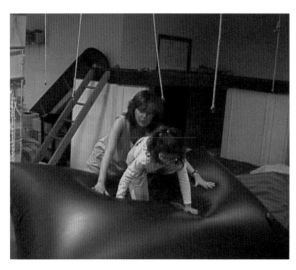

Fig. 3-9
Encourage more mature righting and equilibrium reactions on three dimensionally unstable surfaces.

Postural Intervention Strategies

Play on surfaces that are three dimensional and unstable (such as a therapy ball, hippity hop, large air mattress, truck inner tubes, water bed mattress and large pillows) promotes postural organization. Play wrestling or roughhousing enhances more organized postural responses. These activities can also help to improve respiratory depth and control (see respiratory section).

Playing closer to the ground requires more antigravity strength. The use of movement, as in change in head position in all planes, deep pressure input from a support surface (body, equipment, floor, Figs. 3-9 to 3-15), joint input from weight bearing and muscle input from working against resistance will often add the just right combination of input at the right intensity to facilitate antigravity responses. For these movement experiences to remain organizing, they must be varied. They should incorporate changes in speed, changes in direction, changes in arc of motion, bumps and start-stop sequences and be purposeful and meaningful.

When engaging in these activities it is critical to remember some of the key principles of postural organization. Balance flexion with extension in movement patterns. Pay attention to the jaw, shoulders and hips and watch for any postural fixing. This can usually be seen in patterns of movement at the end of the range such as extreme ab/adduction or flexion/ extension at the shoulders and hips, locking at the elbows, jaw clenching or retraction, cheek retraction, tongue thrust or retraction. These patterns block the active use of muscles down the center of the body as well as dynamic cocontraction patterns around the joints.

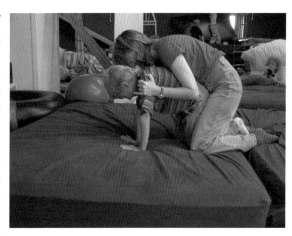

Fig. 3-10

The child with poorly organized postural patterns often initiates many of his or her movements with extension of the neck, back and extremities. This will block the use of more mature patterns and inhibit deeper diaphragmatic breathing. The therapist can work to position him or herself in a way that keeps a small container around the child and facilitate weight bearing through the shoulders and hips (Figs. 3-10 and 3-11) followed by flexion with rotation (Figs. 3-12 to 3-15). Pillows, lycra hung from four points of suspension, body socks, cloth tunnels and large pillows may also be helpful tools in providing a smaller container and inhibiting the unbalanced use of extension.

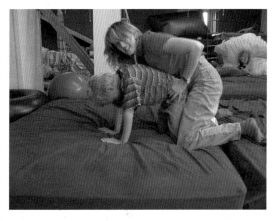

Fig. 3-11

To facilitate and promote cocontraction around the jaw, use oral motor supports which promote biting, tugging and chewing. Resistive sucking may also help promote movement of the jaw, lips and tongue in three-dimensional patterns. To activate shoulders and hips work to facilitate active weight bearing with alignment, keep the body low to the ground and use the upper extremities in heavy work pushing and pulling patterns. It may be necessary to use passive compression and traction to help activate more balanced activity around the joints. Joint compression will facilitate cocontraction patterns and joint traction will help to facilitate more balanced use of flexion.

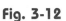

Fig. 3-12

Promote changes in head position in order to stimulate the vestibular system. Adding resistance to the movement will help the child organize the sensation received from body movement, recruit more muscle fibers for building strength and facilitate integration of the new movement patterns into the child's inherent repertoire of purposeful, skilled movement patterns. Avoid giving re-

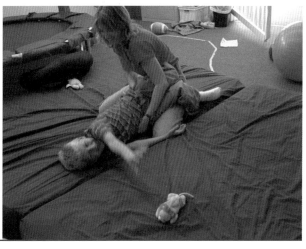

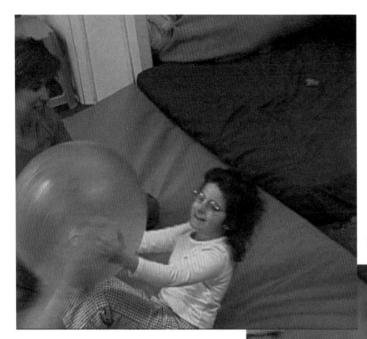

sistance to uncoordinated patterns. It is often more effective to apply resistance in a pattern of apply, hold, release, rather than applying a steady pull or push. Using resistance against total patterns of movement increases sensory input.

Facilitate rotation and counter rotation around midline through work on unstable surfaces (as above or adding shaving cream to an other-

Fig. 3-13

wise more stable surface) positioning, handling, rolling with the child, encouraging the child to use twisting, turning and pulling movements to emerge from small spaces such as under pillows or a small space created by the therapist's body during roughhouse play.

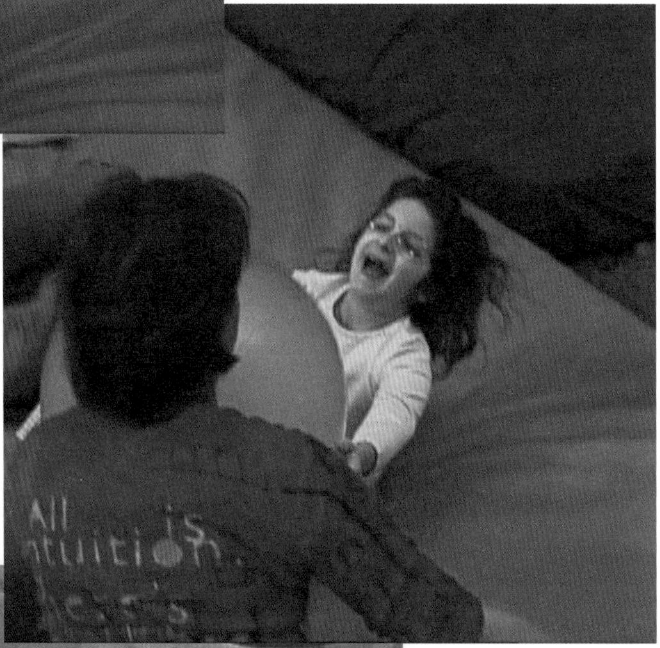

Fig. 3-14

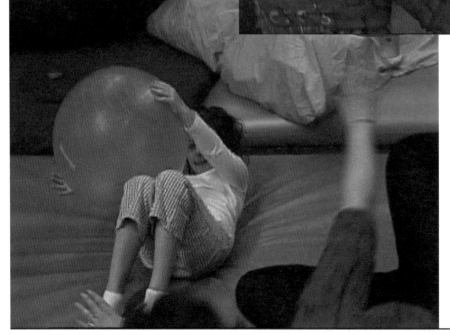

Fig. 3-15

Respiratory Intervention Strategies

When a Therapeutic Listening program is used to address issues with sensory modulation and self regulation it is critical to address any underlying issues of inefficient respiratory patterns. Inability to grade respiratory rate and depth contributes to challenges with modulation, behavioral escalation and self regulation. In individuals who exhibit these difficulties, respiration tends to be short, shallow and often arrhythmical, with periods of breath-holding. Short, shallow breathing patterns obligate the nervous system to a high alert state. In this heightened state, it becomes more challenging to grade responses to stimuli in the environment.

It is important to decrease any postural fixing or breath holding prior to working on deeper respiration. This can be done initially though play on three dimensionally unstable surfaces and roughhouse play.

Many of the activities, positions, handling and sound games mentioned below may be incorporated into or used following activities such as play wrestling, play on an air or water bed mattress, hippity hop or trampoline (sitting, hands and knees are recommended positions of play). Roughhouse play is also best on the ground, i.e. crawling, rolling, moving against the resistance of another person's body, using obstacles created with large, over pillows, inner tubes or large therapy balls, lycra body suits, long knit cloth tunnels etc.

Positioning in relative antigravity flexion will set up the muscles of respiration for optimal biomechanical advantage. Several handling techniques may also be helpful in encouraging deeper breathing patterns.

Fig. 3-16

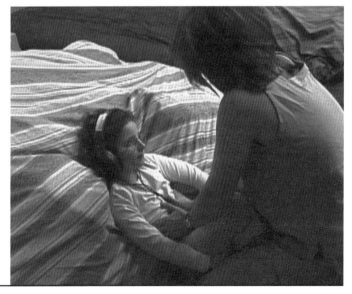

With hands on the side of the ribs gently rock or shake the rib cage in a downward direction toward the child's pelvis (Fig. 3-16). The gentle rocking or shaking helps to further decrease muscle tightness and breath holding. Pay attention to the child's breath while you are doing so. Downward movement of the rib cage goes with exhalation, and it is often helpful to encourage the child to play with vocalization, such as a gentle humming sound, during the action.

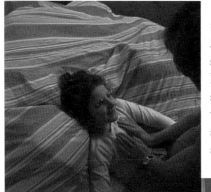

Gently tapping on the muscles of the rib cage may also wake up and prepare them to work in a more efficient manner (Figs. 3-17 to 3-19). The ribs are located just below the clavicles and attach to the sternum in the front and the spine in the back. Make sure to tap along the front of the chest, along both sides and along the ribs and down the spine. This can also be done with a small pliable ball (Gertie® or toss balls work well). This activity often stimulates vocalization. Play with and encourage any sound the child makes!

Figs. 3-17, 18, 19

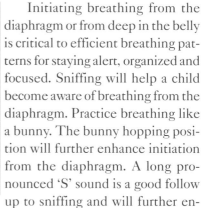

Initiating breathing from the diaphragm or from deep in the belly is critical to efficient breathing patterns for staying alert, organized and focused. Sniffing will help a child become aware of breathing from the diaphragm. Practice breathing like a bunny. The bunny hopping position will further enhance initiation from the diaphragm. A long pronounced 'S' sound is a good follow up to sniffing and will further encourage the use of diaphragmatic breathing. This can be enhanced if done while using the arms to push against a large ball, or the extended arms of another person. Make sure that the child does not pull up the shoulders or lock elbows. Try it while slithering along the floor like a snake.

Extending exhalation is the best way to deepen the breath. Insert a long straw or piece of rubber tubing in a dish tub, or large plastic container filled one quarter full of water with a few drops of dish soap. Encourage the child to grade a long, slow breath to create a bubble monster or volcano that comes to the top and starts to escape the pan or erupt.

Several commercially available kazoos and whistles are also very helpful. Make sure that the piece that goes in the child's mouth is a good fit and encourages a tight seal with the tongue, cheeks and lips.

Fig. 3-20

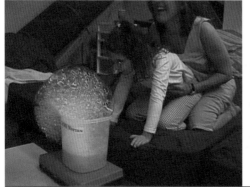

During blowing activities, gentle handling by following the child's breath with the hands may be helpful. Place hands over the lower borders of the ribs along the child's sides just above the waistline. Begin by just 'listening' with your hands, notice and watch for any changes in the movement of the ribs out to the side and slightly upward on the inhale and down toward the floor and in toward the middle on the exhale. Pressure may be increased slightly if immediate change is not evident. Remember to follow the movement of the rib cage.

Specific activities for enhancing respiration might include:

♦ Having the child lie on his stomach and use a straw to blow a ping-pong ball or cotton ball across a room.

♦ Playing catch with bubbles with another person by blowing bubbles to someone, having them catch the bubbles on a wand, blow them back and repeating the cycle. (Blow, catch, blow, catch, etc.)

♦ Volleying bubbles back and forth to another person by isolating and blowing a specific bubble.

♦ Buying gooze or silly goo, placing it on the end of a straw and seeing how big of a bubble can be blown.

♦ Blowing through a string pipe and moving one hand in and out through the circle that is formed by the string.

♦ Blowing a ball pipe and seeing how many times the ball can be caught, how high the ball can be blown and still be caught, how long the ball can be suspended in the air, etc.

♦ Having contests with the child using different blow toys. How long can he or she blow? How loud can he blow? How soft can he or she blow? How many sounds can he or she make on one breath? Can he repeat a rhythm back to you when blowing or have a conversation using whistles or kazoos?

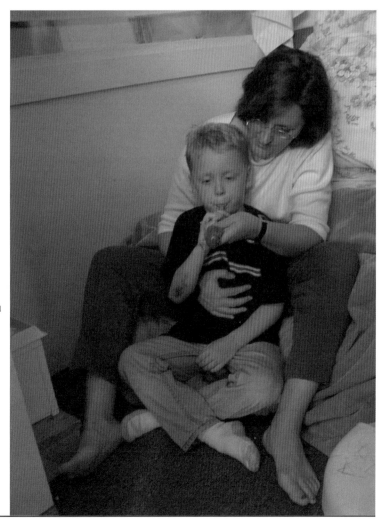

Refinement of Initial Treatment Protocol

Following implementation of an Initial Listening Protocol, refinement of a Therapeutic Listening program should be based upon programming for the area which continues to be the most problematic or has the most global negative impact for the client. Working from the broadest areas to the most specific will promote the most comprehensive change and allow for ever-increasing levels of refinement and organization. Each CD selected in the progression of a listening program should provide more refinement, more precision, greater organization and more finely tuned skill. See page 3-91 for a clinical reasoning model.

Vestibular/Body/ Postural

The use of Carulli initially aides in establishing a body midline, the ability to sustain active postural responses on stable as well as dynamic surfaces as well as an increase in cocontraction patterns and the emergence of rotation and bilateral movements. To further refine these patterns into bilateral skill, facilitate and improve praxis as well as fine motor skill the music that may have the greatest impact is:

Live in Catalunya (Chamber) (04)
Cadaques Night (05)
Nocturne (21)

Oral/Respiratory

The CDs in this category have been known to specifically facilitate increased coordination of the suck/swallow/breath synchrony and respiration. This sensorimotor pattern refers to the timing and interaction among sucking, swallowing and breathing that is available to the infant at birth as a primary mechanism for organizing (arousal, postural development and psychosocial development) and eating. As the baby uses the synchrony the motor patterns become more refined and contribute to a broad range of skills (see Appendix p. 3-73 to 3-75).

Classic (01) for coordination of suck/swallow/breathe
Live in Catalunya (Chamber) (04) for modulation of respiration

Self Regulation/Refined Sensory Modulation

Modulation refers to the ability to organize and process sensory information. This is ultimately tied to self regulation: the ability to achieve, maintain and change state to be able to attend and focus in a manner that matches the demands of the situation (environment/task). As modulation and self regulation emerge and begin to develop (as seen by improvements in sleep/wake cycle, reduction in sensory defensive behaviors, increased regularity of hunger and thirst as well as bowel and bladder function), then the next group of CDs which may be helpful in this area may assist in continued smoothing out of mood variance;

broadening the range of functional arousal states; improving transitions; accepting change and novelty introduced into routines and increasing ability to maintain and adapt level of focus and attention.

Live in Catalunya (Chamber) (04)
Cadaques Night (05)
Nocturne (21)
Cantabile (22)

Sequencing/Timing

Sequencing and timing refers to finer timing in social interaction (i.e. turn taking, response time, etc.), sequencing of thoughts for spoken and written language, the ability to follow multistep directions, motor execution (praxis) and the ability to understand the finer timing and sequencing that is involved in mathematical skills.

Live in Catalunya (Chamber) (04)
Mozart & Contemporaries (08)

Language

Language includes multiple components such as: more accurate and concise expression to interact with others, increased amount and quality of verbal expression, greater ability to attach language to emotions, an increase in the ability to use language to describe and attach meaning to situations, etc.

Classic (01)
Romantic (02)
Mozart & Contemporaries (08)
Nocturne (21)
Cantabile (22)
Lascia Ch'io Pianga (23)

Expression/Emotionality/Engagement

The music on these CDs tends to be more emotionally laden and facilitates broader ranges of affective expression and engagement. This music may also assist an individual to be more tuned into his or her emotions and better able to express himself or herself appropriately, with vocal intonation, speech content and postural cues and gestures.

Romantic (02)
Lascia Ch'io Pianga (23)

Academics

School performance in areas related to reading, writing and mathematics.

Live in Catalunya (Chamber) (04)
Mozart & Contemporaries (08)

Syn-Energy

The concept of Syn-Energy is based on mechanisms that influence the brain and promote states of relaxation and openness to new ideas and learning. These CDs contain natural complex resonance patterns and slight spectral activation for promoting deep relaxation and hemispheric synchronization. This series of CDs is based on the principle of entrainment, the process of two rhythms developing the same pulse through close proximity to one another. Through sound it is possible to influence the rhythmic pulsing of the electrical activity of the brain, thus influencing the level of consciousness and learning associated with the particular brain wave frequency (see box at left).

Brain Wave Frequencies:

Delta - (slow firing; 0.5 to 3 CPS) deep dreamless, sleep, very deep breathing, slow heart rate, cool body temperature

Theta - (4 to 7 CPS mainly in temporal & parietal regions of the brain) unconscious sleep state, deep meditation, deep creative dreams, deep creative thought

Alpha - (8 to 12 CPS brain idle or midpoint, Cool, 1999) (a state less available to children with sensory modulation, attention and learning difficulties) a state of relaxation, daydreaming, creative imagination, connection to subconscious, information synthesis, first assimilation, integrated learning states

Beta - (13 to 40 CPS most commonly recorded in frontal and parietal lobe) logical thought processing, analysis, active, organizational skills, productivity, attention, external focus

High Beta - (over 23 CPS) anxiety, anger, short/shallow breathing

Specific frequency patterns are embedded in specially selected recordings of music and nature sounds. These sound patterns are known as beat frequencies. Two slightly out of sync frequency patterns are presented to each ear through headphones. The difference between the two patterns creates a third frequency pattern as the brain puts together the two frequency patterns that it hears. For example, if an individual listening to a tone that is vibrating at 440 hertz (Hz) in one ear and one at 448 Hz in the other ear, a third frequency of 8 Hz will be produced. The 8 Hz pulse has the potential to synchronize the brain waves to 8 Hz, a pattern in the alpha range.

In addition when these electrical signals occur with relatively equal frequency and strength in both hemispheres they create a synchronization of the two sides of the brain. This synchronization sets the stage for listening and learning.

The idea of beat frequencies is not new. Robert Monroe and the Monroe Institute have worked for years researching the effects of these specially embedded signals in white noise and Music, a process known as Hemi-Sync®.

In Syn-Energy, Steinbach has created a new technology, frequency-space-time shifts, that allows the integration of these signals for hemisphere synchronization and deep relaxation to be created and integrated into the natural spectrum of music and nature sounds.

For example in the *Mysteries of Water (CS 931)*, a third frequency pattern is created when the two xylophones are played at slightly different pitches and are played in the right and left channels. This is coupled with the sounds of water and music that are played at about 50–70 beats per minute. All of these factors have the potential to entrain alpha, a quiet alert state associated with modulation, attention, relaxation and learning.

This process of relaxation and hemispheric synchronization helps the individual transition more smoothly and easily through different behavioral states.

Following these same concepts, *Nature Sound Synergy (CS 933)* utilizes the sound of the incoming surf on two sides of a peninsula, slightly out of sync. Two Tibetan bowls that are played at two slightly different pitches are recorded into the right and left channels creating a third frequency matrix. This third sound matrix along with other music and natural sound patterns entrains the listener to the deeply relaxed state of theta.

The use of the Syn-Energy CDs creates an external source that makes it possible to drive the electrical firing of the brain. They support an individual to shift efficiently from one state of consciousness to another. They can be used alone or as a part of an ongoing Therapeutic Listening program. *Mysteries of Water* is often used with individuals in a state associated with anxiety and/or compulsive and habitual behavior. Since alpha is the quiet alert state, or the brain's idle state, training alpha appears to help many such individuals shift into a state where more flexible and creative behavioral strategies can be accessed. This CD has been helpful in training many children who have difficulty grading arousal levels, i.e. those who overshoot the middle and run in high gear.

Nature Sound Synergy and *Alpha and Omega (CS 932)* are used to promote relaxation in terms of stress and pain management. Many therapists have used them as part of other therapeutic regimes such as craniosacral, myofascial therapy and relaxation training.

CD Descriptions

CS 931 - Mystery of Water

The music on this CD is skillfully combined with the sounds of water producing a heightened spatial awareness for the listener. The spectral activation is similar to SAMONAS SE recordings. The frequency displacement ranges from frequencies that correspond to alpha state with some in the neighboring theta region. This CD may be used to facilitate an alpha state in the listener. This has been used for children and adults who demonstrate difficulties with anxiety and compulsive behavior. There is a slight lateralization as the listener senses the water moving back and forth between the right and left ears. This is hypothesized to support the communication between right and left hemispheres which appears to enhance attention, sensory awareness and modulation, as well as intuitive processing. This may also be used by the therapist to enhance relaxation, creativity and development of intuitive clinical reasoning abilities.

CS 932 - Alpha and Omega

This recording combines sounds of nature with harmonics which resonate at the same frequency as the earth, sun and stars. Track 1 entrains the listener into the theta state. This may be useful for encouraging deep relaxation and integration of newly learned materials. One must be careful in using this CD with individuals with attention difficulties as recent research shows that many who experience difficulties with attention have an over abundance of theta activity. Track 2 takes the listener deeper into a delta state.

CS 933 - Nature Sound Synergy

The sound on this CD is the combination of music, nature sounds and the Tibetan sound bowl which resonates with the vibrations of the Sun and Jupiter. Like *Alpha and Omega*, Track 1 is in the theta domain and Track 2 takes the listener into the deepest state of relaxation through entraining the listener into the delta frequency. Many therapists have found this helpful in working with clients for profound states of relaxation and pain management.

Basic Equipment Needs for
Therapeutic Listening

CD Player*

Most portable CD players are adequate for the purpose of Therapeutic Listening. When shopping for a CD player, bring the headphones which will be used for listening and a familiar CD. Plug the headphones in to the headphone jack. Turn the volume up to a relatively loud level then gradually turn the volume down to a soft level. As the volume decreases, the sound should remain equal in both ears. At quieter volumes, make sure neither the right or left channel is lost, nor the balance shifted to one side or the other.

When listening through the headphones, no background hissing, crackling, popping, or other distortions should be audible. CD players need to have a random play or shuffle feature to ensure the random nature preferred in Therapeutic Listening programs. When using a portable CD player, it is preferable to use batteries rather than plugging the CD player into an electrical socket. Use of an outside power source comes with the certainty of picking up unwanted electrical distortion and "dirt."

Headphones**

Headphones need to be good quality with a high resistance or impedance of at least 150 Ohms and a frequency sensitivity to 23,000 Hz.

Headphones should be circumaural with an open ear system. The circumaural (or shell type) creates enough space around the ear (sounds need to travel through an air cushion to keep the sensitive portion of the inner ear from being overwhelmed). The open ear system maintains appropriate perception and auditory-figure ground.

Headphones with volume controls to either ear are not appropriate because the transmission of lower frequencies may be poor. This may also shift the volume weight to one ear which may also be inappropriate.

Setting the Volume***

Place the headphones on your own ears. Set the volume at a comfortable level. You should be able to carry on a conversation without raising your voice. If the individual wearing the headphones requests the volume to be either raised or lowered, this is appropriate as long as he/she can still engage in a conversation without raising his/her voice. If you follow this rule of thumb, the volume will remain at an appropriate level.

Audio tape technology is not used for therapeutic purposes because it generally only captures frequencies up to 16,000 Hz. Frequencies beyond 16,000 Hz are critical for maintaining attention and providing the finer details about the sound source.

** Due to the spatial aspects and the right ear weighting of the recordings, it is critical to place the headphones on the correct ears as designated on the Sennheiser headphones. Do not reverse the headphones because it confuses the spatial quality of the recordings.*

*** If it is possible to use a decibel reader, one can set the volume very accurately between 45 and 55 dB.*

Implementation of Therapeutic Listening Programs for Clinic, Home and School Environments

When choosing the environment in which a Therapeutic Listening program should occur, it is important to consider a number of factors. All of these factors must be considered in order to maximize the outcomes obtained from a Therapeutic Listening program. The most important question to ask may be "What is possible?" What is possible will vary for each individual and each family. Consistency of listening is primary; listening should occur at least 5 days per week to be most effective.

CLINIC

Therapeutic Listening as an in-clinic program is possibly the least desired approach in most circumstances. It is unusual that a client would be seen at a clinic frequently enough to obtain optimum results from a Therapeutic Listening program. The clinic environment provides an opportunity to explore the suitability of using a Therapeutic Listening program and observe the client's response to different discs. However, once this assessment is completed, the listening itself most typically occurs in other environments.

There are exceptions to this routine. Sometimes families or individual clients elect a treatment intensive as a model for intervention. During a treatment intensive, a client may be seen 1 or 2 times daily for a period of 3-5 days. Clients may then continue with a home program.

Additionally, in a rare number of instances, the client takes a longer than expected time to accommodate to the headphones. In this situation, it is important to persist in the clinic rather than send the client home with this as a continued challenge. Rarely do headphones remain challenging longer than one treatment session. In the situations where headphones remain an issue, it is important to muster all possible resources to support the child/client and family through the process of accepting headphones. Persistence with headphones should only occur if it is what the family chooses. The therapist must also believe that Therapeutic Listening is important for the child/client as the therapist's beliefs will greatly impact the success of the program. Doubts, fears or concerns on the therapist's part will be conveyed to the client. The therapist's entire demeanor, even if it is necessary to physically hold headphones on a crying, struggling child, must be calm, kind, gentle and assured. If everyone is united in the belief that listening is important for the child, then wearing headphones should not be presented as a choice. The therapist's language must communicate this intent to the child. "It is time to do listening now" carries a different message than "Would you like to do some listening?" It is also important to validate the child's feelings about the headphones while not giving the child the idea that the headphones are a choice. "This feels so hard right now" acknowledges the child's fear, confusion or upset while not relenting on the importance of persistence. The child can have active choices around other activities to do while listening; listening should not be conveyed as a choice.

The other circumstance around which an in-clinic listening program is probably the most appropriate choice is when a program is being selected for a child whose history suggests a pattern of extreme sensitivity or reactivity any time the conditions for change within the nervous system are created. Though sometimes treatment outcomes eventually seem positive, the child may have experienced a period of extreme disorganization that was frightening both to the child and to the child's family. If the potential for disorganization seems great, then treatment should begin within the clinic where it is possible to support the child and the child's family fully and make appropriate program modifications in an ongoing manner.

HOME

Once a family has been trained in the use of Therapeutic Listening, home is probably the ideal environment in which listening can occur. Typically, it is simple to incorporate listening into daily routines. Always, the family is well-versed in minute changes in the child's behavior and can request assistance for program modification as needed.

When Therapeutic Listening is done as a home program, it is important not to jeopardize the effectiveness of the program by compromising on the quality of the equipment used or by decreasing listening times to less than what is deemed appropriate.

A method of follow up is critical to positive outcomes. If the therapist supervising changes in the program doesn't see the child regularly, a concrete form of communication needs to be in place.

Home Program Supports

Home Therapeutic Listening programs typically follow the guidelines previously delineated. The following suggestions may be helpful when implementing a Therapeutic Listening program at home.

♦ Listening during breakfast seems to fit well within most families' daily routines.

♦ Often after school time provides another suitable listening time.

♦ Listening close to bed time should be avoided until the impact of the CDs is understood on the individual.

♦ If the child does not have a history of motion sickness, listening while riding in the car is another possibility. Use a portable CD player and headphones only. Never use the car stereo system.

♦ Provision of a variety of novel media for artistic self-expression (markers, stampers, finger paints, clay, crayons, water colors, Blopens®) can be useful supplementary activities while listening.

♦ Provision of a variety of novel toys for tactile exploration (squeeze balls, Koosh® balls, squirt toys, bean play, bean bags, hand toys, puzzles) may also be helpful.

♦ Provision of a variety of respiratory activities (straws, blow toys, whistles, kazoos, bubble toys) is another possibility for supporting listening.

♦ Posture should be appropriately supported during longer listening times (bean bag chair, therapy ball, swing).

♦ Sometimes it is helpful to use a tune belt and have the individual listen while walking or on a small riding toy or being pulled in a wagon. Active bicycle riding while listening is **not** recommended, however, the child might ride on an attachment to an adult's bicycle while listening.

SCHOOL

Therapeutic Listening can also occur effectively within in a school setting if it is possible for the student to listen at least 5 days per week. This degree of consistency should not compromise overall results. Therapeutic Listening within an educational setting can occur in a variety of manners - in individual therapy sessions, in resource rooms, or in the regular education classroom. The most important factor may be that those helping to implement the Therapeutic Listening program understand the behaviors (both desired and undesired) that are being targeted and will reliably document results.

Setting Up Listening Therapy Programs in the Schools

There is no wrong or right to any of the models proposed. The circumstances of each situation and the conviction of those implementing the program will dictate what is possible. It is important to attempt the **most intensive level of intervention** that is possible. That will necessitate sharing responsibilities for listening programs with other school personnel so that programs can be carried out on a daily basis rather than only when a therapist is available.

One possible model is that of a listening lab or listening stations. In this situation, a resource classroom might be used as the listening station and programs might be implemented and monitored by a resource teacher. Students could listen daily during time already spent in the resource room. The resource teacher could determine appropriate activities for each student to complete during listening time.

Other therapists have found use of a listening lab challenging and have elected to use Therapeutic Listening in the schools only as part of the students' occupational therapy programs. While less optimal, therapists have had success providing Therapeutic Listening for individual students only during school therapy sessions.

The following page contains a model that was successfully implemented in several school districts.

Suggested sequence of events

♦ In-service on listening (60-90 minutes) provided to full school staff.

♦ In-service on listening provided to families.

♦ Following the in-service, support solicited for equipment from special education director.

♦ Individual follow-up with classroom teachers regarding willingness to use Therapeutic Listening in the classroom as part of a student's daily classroom routine.

♦ Appropriate students on OT case load assessed for Therapeutic Listening programs.

♦ Follow-up with teachers regarding any differences in students' behaviors following initial assessment and use of discs.

♦ Parent permission to implement a Therapeutic Listening program for each individual student acquired.

♦ Equipment needed to support the number of students assessed presented to special education director.

♦ Assignment of strategic geographic locations of listening stations within classrooms; CD players and discs remain within the classroom; a listening schedule is created for students (some in this classroom, some in nearby classrooms) to use equipment at a designated time each day.

♦ A short list of appropriate questions for each student created for home room teachers to complete at the end of each week to monitor progress on listening programs and determine needs for changes. Questions would be applicable to school and reflect reasons a particular child was on a listening program (i.e. Improvements in handwriting? Improvements in attention? Improvements in independence in work? Improvements in ability to follow directions?).

♦ Encouragement for other school staff to become trained in the use of Therapeutic Listening by attending a full workshop so that responsibility for monitoring programs could be shared.

Questions Frequently Asked By Therapists

How is the music modified?

The music on the Therapeutic Listening CDs is modified in several different ways, depending upon the CD being used.

♦ Modified CDs (i.e. *Ease Disc, Mozart—Modified*) - the music on these CDs is processed through an alternating high pass low pass filter. Sometimes the higher frequencies are allowed to pass; sometimes the lower frequencies are allowed to pass. This type of modification is referred to as modulation and is what creates the disrupted sound to the music. Modulation works at the level of the middle ear, helping to restore or enhance the range of biomechanical flexibility of the middle ear muscles and exercising the relax/contract (monitor/focus) capacities of the middle ear. Flexibility of these muscles is necessary to transmit sensory information to primary sensory processing centers that support sensory modulation, vestibular postural organization and integration and social/cognitive function.

♦ SAMONAS - CQ (*Classic Quality*) CDs are naturally spectrally activated. They are selections of classical music that are recorded to the specifications of Ingo Steinbach with respect to instrumentation and preservation of the space within which the recording occurs (see SONAS description, p. 3-19). HS (*Healing Sounds*) CDs have dampened frequencies below 300 Hz. SE and ST SAMONAS recordings undergo a process that increases the level of spectral activation. When passages of the music are spectrally activated, it means that the harmonics in the higher frequencies have been intensified. It is in the higher harmonic ranges that the detailed information of sound is carried (i.e. the information that allows one to perceive the differences between two female voices). Spectral activation does not create a disrupted quality to the overall sound of the music. Additionally, some selections on ST SAMONAS CDs are known as high extension passages. These are brief passages of music where only the high harmonics remain; the overall volume of these passages of music will seem quite soft and the ears will have to reach for the sound.

At what volume should listening occur?

A decibel reading of 45-55 dB for listening is well within OSHA standards. A decibel reader can give precise readings as to the listening volume. However, a general rule of thumb is that the listener should not be speaking in a louder than typical voice for carrying on a conversation. If he/she does seem to be speaking loudly, the volume is probably too high and should be decreased.

Can listening be done over loudspeakers?

Once loudspeakers are used, the listening program being delivered is radically different. Sound travels as waves through space. The greater the space through which the sound waves must travel, the less the sound waves impact the listener. The modified CDs and most SAMONAS CDs are NOT configured for speaker use. They should only be used over headphones. Of the SAMONAS CDs, only the CQ (Classic Quality) level of recordings are configured for speaker use and can be played as background music in a classroom to promote general organization, to help with transitions, to create group attention, or to facilitate motor fluidity during a handwriting group. It is not recommended that the CQ CDs be used over speakers as a true Therapeutic Listening program for an individual.

Rarely, when headphones are not appropriate for use because of the child's age (under two years of age), the modified CDs may be used over speakers. If this is the case, the speakers should be of good quality, the child should be relatively stationary with respect to the speakers and should be positioned in the apex of the triangle formed between the speakers and the child, and the room in which listening occurs should be fairly small. A bathroom might be a good choice.

What activities should be discouraged while listening to the CDs?

Generally, any activities that make the child seem unavailable are not recommended during listening. TV, videos, computer use and video games are all discouraged except as activities of last resort. Additionally, while it is usually fine for a child to play with cars or other favorite toys, the child should be using these toys in a constructive or creative manner. Lining up toys or other objects would be an activity to discourage during listening.

Is there a standard progression of CDs for a Therapeutic Listening program?

A basic beginning protocol is recommended for most clients. This protocol includes 2 - 12 weeks of modulated music (i.e. *EASe, Rhythm & Rhyme, Kidz Jamz, Mozart for Modulation* - Modified, *Baroque for Modulation* - Modified, *Mozart String Quartets I & II*) followed by implementation of SAMONAS. *Carulli* (in a level of activation appropriate for the client) is the most frequent CD to follow modulated music though *Sounds of Nature* may be the next CD for others. If issues are more body-related, then *Carulli* is the logical next step. If issues are related to spatial awareness, then *Sounds of Nature* may be the appropriate choice. In almost all cases, modulated music is followed by use of *Carulli* and *Sounds of Nature* before other SAMONAS CDs are introduced. This basic protocol ensures the maximum effectiveness of a Therapeutic Listening program for individuals whose issues include sensory modulation/sensory integration difficulties.

How long should a client remain on modulated music?

The greater the degree of difficulties with sensory modulation, the longer a client will remain on modulated music. If a client has a history of extreme reactivity to a variety of sensory input and has difficulty with basic physiological regulation (wake/sleep, appetite cycles, bladder control, etc.), the client will likely remain on modulated music for 10-12 weeks before any other CDs are introduced. Even at 10-12 weeks, modulated music may remain in the client's Therapeutic Listening program for at least one session per day. During this 10-12 week period, no one CD will be used for a period of time longer than 3 weeks. Variety within the modulated music range is important to ensure that habituation and routinization do not occur. Clients with less significant modulation disorders will remain on modulated music for a shorter duration. Clients with minimal modulation issues or with a history of chronic ear infections might remain on modulated music only 2-3 weeks.

We started listening and my client seems to have increased auditory sensitivity. What does this mean?

The most primitive defensive response is to shut-off sensation. Often times, when children with sensory defensiveness begin a Therapeutic Listening program, they cover their ears, begin to complain of noise, etc. These are all higher levels of adaptive behavior than shutting off. Children will typically progress through this phase to an even more advanced level of processing auditory input reflected by the ability to grade their response to sound, such as an increased attentiveness and connectedness in more complex sound environments. Again, increased auditory sensitivity can be a positive adaptive response. However, if auditory sensitivity with negative responses persists for more than 1-2 weeks, consider modifying listening times, CDs, or overall sensory diet strategies.

Why listen at home instead of the clinic?

The goal for a Therapeutic Listening program is consistency. Consistency in listening is what will promote the most efficient, effective change. The most positive and long-lasting results will be gained when the program is able to be implemented on a daily basis. However, clinic programs may be beneficial initially when a child has difficulty acclimating to listening or where additional problem solving regarding therapeutic support is needed.

Additionally, if a client has a history of extreme disregulation and has become disorganized each time change has been introduced into his/her life, then an in-clinic intensive is recommended prior to implementation of listening at home. The intensive should last a minimum of 5 days, preferably 2 sessions per day.

How do I know when to change a child's Therapeutic Listening program?

Change a child's program when you stop seeing benefit, when you want to add the next level of refinement or when the child indicates a need for a change (boredom, etc.). In general, a child should not remain on a Therapeutic Listening program without some change to the music for longer than 2-3 weeks. While it is not unusual for a child to listen for 6 months or longer, there should have been many changes to the child's program during this interval.

How do I work through getting headphones on a child who is resistant to wearing them?

Typically, the novelty of the headphones rather than the actual feel of the headphones or the sound of the music is what is upsetting to the child. Therefore, it is important to gently persist through the period of upset, using whatever distractions or other means possible to help keep the headphones on. However, persistence should only occur with full permission of parents. If it is known in advance that a child for whom headphones will be challenging is coming for a listening program, solicit the support of your colleagues for this session. It is truly important to persist; if you only work up to the hard part and then remove the headphones, the hard part is never done. A pattern of learned resistance is developed and the child never gets to experience the potential benefits of a Therapeutic Listening program. Possibly the single most important factor in helping a child with headphones is the therapist's belief that wearing headphones can occur - that it is possible.

Will wireless headphones work?

No. Wireless headphones have a low dynamic frequency (range of response). The quality, especially of the upper frequencies in which the important discriminative information is carried, is lost. Wireless headphones also pick up unwanted higher frequencies from any other electronic appliances that are being used within a nearby space.

When the child listens, he/she looks great. When we remove the headphones, the child doesn't seem to hold the changes. What should I do?

Therapeutic Listening cannot exist in a vacuum. It will be

important to solidify any skills boosted or facilitated by listening with all of the other tools in your therapy tool box. Therapeutic Listening may open the window for emergent skill; however, then you must go through that open window with everything else available to you and possible for the child. One particular key element in intervention is that of postural activation. Postural activation, organization and refinement of core movement patterns seems to be the 'glue' which helps changes hastened by listening to hold. (See section Postural Control, p. 3-42). If sensory defensiveness is present it must be addressed vigorously.

I have heard that *Carulli* might intensify compulsive or rigid behaviors in children. Is this true?

This occasionally does happen; however, it should not be considered a 'blanket rule' to avoid *Carulli* with children who are rigid or compulsive. Rather, implement a program with *Carulli* if it seems to be a match for the child's motor issues. While the child is on *Carulli*, carefully monitor for any increase in undesired behaviors that last more than 2-3 days. In this situation, it may be best to avoid use of *Carulli* for periods longer than 3-4 weeks total.

Can a child begin a Therapeutic Listening program if they have PE* tubes?

Many children who have PE tubes have benefitted from Therapeutic Listening. PE tubes are usually inserted into the less flexible portion of the eardrum, thus having little effect on its movement.

PE tubes are often inserted into the tympanic membrane (eardrum) to drain fluid which has built up in the middle ear. The procedure is typically used for children with recurrent ear infection or who have fluid build up due to allergies.

What do I do if I have difficulties?

♦ Inconsistent listening times - this is a compromise; the program is most effective if the input can summate; opt for the maximum consistency possible - strive for a home or school program.

♦ Bed wetting - have the child listen earlier in the day; decrease the listening time (if on modulated music, decrease to one session per day; if on SAMONAS, decrease to the amount of time where no difficulties were observed); go to a less intense CD; often the level of activation of the CD is the problem so try a less intense CD as a first strategy.

♦ Sleep disturbances - have the child listen earlier in the day; decrease the listening time (see above); go to a less intense CD.

♦ Emotional liability/behavioral issues - provide sensory diet strategies; decrease listening times (see above); go to a less intense CD, return to modulated music if this has been removed.

* Patchless Eustachian Tubes (PE Tubes)

◆ Stuttering - make sure the headphones are on correctly (red on right); if on ST 103 change to a SAMONAS SE or *Healing Sounds* version of *Carulli*, or to a different CD.

How do I Know if My Therapeutic Listening program is "*just right*"?

Your Therapeutic Listening Program is probably "*just right*" when:

◆ the client is making changes.
◆ changes are occurring in the targeted areas (modulation, mediation of postural tone, postural attention, motor control, spatial-temporal organization, communication).
◆ undesired behaviors exhibited are not outside the bounds of what can be typically exhibited.
◆ mild stress may be present but isn't enough to create extreme disorganization.
◆ sensory strategies that have worked in the past continue to be effective for reorganization.

Your Therapeutic Listening Program is probably "*too much*" when:

◆ the client's typical daily rhythms (sleep, appetite) are disrupted for more than a day or two.
◆ the degree of disorganization present is uncomfortable for the client or the client's family.
◆ behavioral shifts interfere with function in other environments (school, home, etc.).

Your Therapeutic Listening Program is probably "*not enough*" when:

◆ there is no increase in energy and ability to sustain an optimal arousal state.
◆ the music doesn't hold client's attention and noncompliance persists.
◆ change noted is minimal and doesn't seem to hold.

You may notice signs of discomfort or tension in clients during the use of Therapeutic Listening Programs. Behaviors such as emotional or physical withdrawal, postural rigidity, shallowness of respiratory patterns and lack of engagement might be observed. However, it is the frequency, intensity and duration with which these behaviors are noted and their interference with functional outcomes that should be used to assess the need to change the Therapeutic Listening Program.

What changes should I look for?

If your Therapeutic Listening program is *"just right"* then you will observe changes in the targeted areas of intervention. These changes might include:

Modulation
- Improvement in sleep/wake cycles.
- Reduction of sensory defensive behaviors.
- A "smoothing out" of mood variance and arousal state.
- Toilet training.
- Cessation of bed wetting.
- Increased regularity of hunger and thirst cycles.
- Improved focus and attention.
- Improvement in transitions.

Postural Tone/Postural Attention/Postural Adaptation
- Establishment of body midline.
- Ability to sustain active posture on stable and dynamic surfaces.
- Improved cocontraction around shoulders and hips.
- Active use of rotation in movement patterns.

Motor Control
- Use of bilateral motor patterns.
- "Emergence" of praxis.
- Improved articulation.
- Improved fine motor skill.

Spatial-Temporal Organization
- Improved timing of motor execution.
- Improved timing of social interactions.
- Discrimination of the dimensionality and directionality of spatial concepts.
- Improved ability to maneuver through space.
- Improved handwriting and visual motor skill.

Communication
- Greater range of nonverbal communication.
- Nonverbal communication matches communicative intent.
- Greater emotional expressiveness.
- Improvement in pragmatic language use.

Treatment Guidelines
Appendix/Forms

Designing a Sensory Diet

Patricia Wilbarger (1984) coined the term 'sensory diet' to explain how certain sensory experiences can be used to enhance occupational performance in any individual as well as contribute to the remediation of developmental and sensory processing disruptions. According to Wilbarger, "sensory diet is not a specific intervention technique. Rather, it is a strategy for developing individualized home programs that are practical, carefully scheduled and based on the concept that controlled sensory input can effect functional abilities" (2001, p. 42).

Implementation of an appropriate sensory diet across all environments is important for individuals on a Therapeutic Listening program and is critical to lasting positive outcomes. Each individual needs certain amounts and types of sensory input or activity each day to be the most alert, adaptable and skillful in performing their everyday activities successfully. Much of the following is based on the work of Patricia Wilbarger and Julia Wilbarger.

Creating a sensory diet of specific activities and strategies helps to sustain an "optimal" level of arousal and enhance an individual's ability to regulate (i.e., keep in a state of balance) his or her own nervous system.

When designing such an activity plan it is important to first ask the question:

"What sensory inputs or strategies does the child seek or use to organize his or her nervous system and keep it focused?"

When asking this question, sensory input in the areas of smell, taste, oral motor requirements, movement, touch, sight and sound all need to be explored.

For any given task, a combination of these various inputs will help support the level of organization needed to perform everyday tasks successfully.

When constructing a sensory diet, it will be important to consider the:
   timing of the sensory input;
   intensity needed; and
   quality of the sensations that will be most organizing for the child's nervous system.

The activity plan may also involve the scheduling of leisure activities that are most organizing.

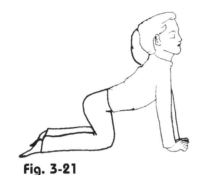

Fig. 3-21

Avoid postures shown here, e.g. hyperextension of the neck, locked joints/ elbows, etc. (See pages. 4-44 through 46).

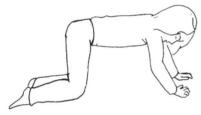

Fig. 3-22

Strive for proper alignment of proximal joints.

Modulators/Activities/Accommodations

♦ **Deep pressure touch** e.g. firm massage, wrapping in heavy blankets, wearing lycra suits

♦ **Proprioception** (i.e., the input to and from joints and muscles) e.g. crashing, holding, lifting, pulling, pushing or jumping with joints in alignment.

♦ **Heavy work** (i.e., a type of proprioception and includes anything that makes the muscles activate against resistance) e.g. rolling, crawling up inclines, climbing, stretching apart bicycle inner tubes, moving furniture, carrying heavy items, roughhouse play. Work toward optimal alignment at jaw, shoulders and hips. It is critical to remember that heavy work is about activation of proximal musculature and that without proper alignment these activities will not be nearly as organizing (Figs. 3-21 & 3-22).

♦ **Movement** e.g. swinging, rocking, dancing, jumping, tumbling, rolling on floor, trampoline games (Note: movement is about moving the head out of the vertical plane). Notice also the qualities of movement e.g. rhythmic movement is often very calming in contrast to fast changeable movement. What kinds of movement does the child currently provide for himself or herself? Can these types of movement be brought into other environments? Experiment with different types of seating and see how those differences affect the child. Do movement breaks help during times of focused attention? How often do they need to be? How long? Does it help the child concentrate during seat work if he or she has been involved in physical activity or movement experiences just prior to doing the work?

♦ **Oral/Motor/Respiratory (Oetter, et al, 1995)** The mouth supports all sensorimotor functions. Activating the mouth has a direct affect on the entire body. What tastes seem to be most organizing to the child? Experiment with intense flavors - sour and spicy tend to be the most alerting. Sucking and chewing may be more calming. Does the child stay appropriately focused on a task better if he or she has some munchies? What kinds of munchies work? Provide those kinds of munchies at times requiring focused attention (e.g. sucking through a straw or on a piece of hard candy; chewing a piece of gum; biting on pretzels or crackers; etc.) Combine the oral motor requirement with the taste that seems most organizing for the child. **Respiration**: Aim to increase depth of breath and decrease rate of respiration. Rapid, short, shallow breathing greatly amplifies difficulties with modulating sensation and sensory defensive/ overload responses. Experiment with resistive sucking activities, blowing activities, breathing activities such as making power sounds (i.e., low sounds from down in the belly, whistle play, kazoo play, blow darts, blowing bubbles into silly goo with straws, using a straw in bath time to blow bubbles).

♦ It may also be helpful to consider what smells support the child's nervous system. Are smells helpful? If so what types of smells? Would the use of certain aroma therapy oils support the child in remaining in an optimum state of arousal e.g., peppermint oil is known to be alerting.

♦ **Sound** Sound can be a powerful modulator. Some sounds are alerting while other sounds are more calming and can create a state of stillness within the nervous system. When considering sound in a sensory diet for the child, it is important to consider what sounds and rhythms support a balanced state in his or her nervous system and what creates a sense of overload. For example, what music seems to most compliment the daily activities the child is needing to perform? What sounds are energizing and alerting to move with? What sounds are more calming and grounding? Does the child need complete silence when focusing? Does music help? If so, what kind? Is the music more organizing if he or she listens to it through headphones?

♦ **Vision** Visual inputs are often used as the sensory snack part of a sensory diet. While not being the most powerful input for nervous system organization, considering the impact of varying visual sensations on the child's nervous system can be helpful in planning a complete sensory diet. What types of visual input are distracting for the child? What kind of lighting or colors seems to help the child concentrate most?

♦ **Environment** The above questions give a starting place for trying to figure out the child's sensory diet. A final aspect to consider is the feel of the overall environment. Does the child attend better sitting at a table to work or lying on the floor? Are small, enclosed places (a nest) more organizing than more wide open spaces? It is important to be aware of what qualities, in an environment, support the child's nervous system and then seek to create those environmental qualities, on a daily basis, for optimal function.

Other considerations when planning a sensory diet

Repetition of Sensory Input
Sensory motor activity must be repeated throughout the day to help the child maintain an optimal level of organization.

For children with sensory defensiveness, recovery from overreactions to sensation is often slow unless specific modulating sensory inputs (sensory diet) are introduced to bring the nervous system back into a state of balance.

Likewise, children who experience difficulty getting their system up out of a low arousal state often need sensory input to bring the nervous system back up into a more optimal arousal state.

Increase predictability of schedule and routines

New activities or change of any type can be very disturbing to individuals with sensory defensiveness. Predictability and preparation decrease the problems. Establish predictability without rigidity so that flexibility is possible.

It is important that the child previews a typical day to prepare for times during that day where organizing sensory input could be scheduled.

Reduce disruptive or disorganizing stimulation in the environment and interactions

It is also important to become aware of those sensations the child will typically avoid or that seem particularly disorganizing to the child. Watching for the subtle signs of avoidance can offer important clues about how the child's nervous system functions.

Sensation that is overwhelming to the child's nervous system will build upon the aversive sensation that went before it. Each sensation builds upon the next eventually leading to a state of overload or shut down. It is therefore critical to notice those aversive sensations, before they build, providing contrasting input that is organizing. It may be helpful for the child to create a hideout area at home that is free from sensory intrusions and that contains those objects and elements that are essentially organizing.

Overview of MORE : Integrating the Mouth with Sensory and Postural Function

At birth the mouth exhibits the most organized sensory integrative and neuromotor behaviors available to the infant. The primary oral motor mechanism is the suck/swallow/breathe (SSB) synchrony. While each component has a distinct function, they are strongly integrated in both automatic and voluntary patterns. It may be most helpful to think of the relationship as synergistic: each element supporting, enhancing and interacting with the other to varying degrees depending on the activity. This synergistic interaction extends throughout life.

The primitive synchrony evolves into synergy as the suck/seal/vacuum component prepares the system for coordinated swallow. Swallowing then sets up change and variation of respiratory rate and depth. Respiratory flexibility then makes it possible to support the suck/swallow components. As each component develops and refines, that refinement contributes to the development and refinement of the other components. Early in development suck is the only oral motor skill that can influence the synergy. Later, bite, crunch, chew and lick followed by suck, seal, vacuum, swallow and respiration become additional ways to access and activate the synergy.

Anatomically, neurologically and biomechanically, the functions of the SSB synchrony/synergy have direct and indirect influences on many aspects of life and human development. As the developmental model illustrates, the influences are neither directional nor mutually exclusive. These interrelationships also imply that we can influence the cycle by addressing the SSB synchrony/synergy and its specific components. Bringing arousal into optimal range, for example, while developing strategies for self regulation (i.e. non-nutritive sucking, deep breaths) may allow better coordination of the SSB for feeding and smiling, vocalizing, etc.

Clinical work has also lead to an awareness of the other aspects of development (throughout life) that may be influenced either positively or negatively by the SSB. The model outlines the relationship between the synchrony/synergy and other developmental processes. The synchrony and its components are so primal that is is easy to take them for granted, but as one studies the foundations of the increasingly complex behaviors identified in the two outer circles of the diagram, it is not surprising that even subtle disruption in any element of the SSB may have a far reaching impact on development and function. The disruption need not originate from the SSB synchrony it-

RELATIONSHIP OF DEVELOPMENT TO THE
SUCK/SWALLOW/BREATHE SYNCHRONY

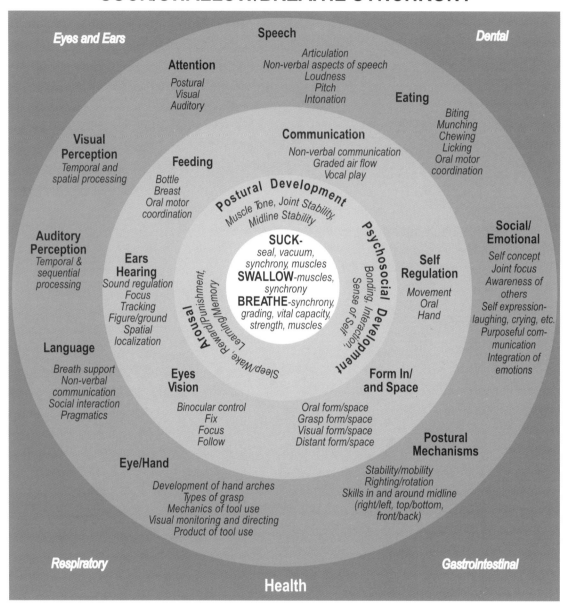

Patricia Oetter, MA, OTR/L, FAOTA © 1989
Oetter, Richter, Frick. revised 1993, 1998

This model is based on the neural construct that structure drives function and function refines and elaborates on structure which in turn refines and elaborates function. The suck/swallow/breathe synchrony lies at the center of this structure/function paradigm for many sensorimotor and developmental functions. Each ring in the diagram represents greater refinement and elaboration of earlier functions.

From: **MORE Integrating the Mouth with Sensory and Postural**
Functions by Oetter, Richter & Frick, 1995. Printed with permission from
PDP Press, Inc., 1137 N. McKusick Road Ln, Stillwater, MN 55082

self, but can derive from other elements that effect it, i.e. muscle tone, neurological problems, disease processes, sensory processing, etc.

Suck/blow/bite/crunch/chew/lick are major components of oral motor activity which can be incorporated into meals and snacks and play activities with food or nonfood items. Use of these components as well as taste, temperature, texture, size and form will help improve and work towards more functional synergy of SSB elements. A general guideline to follow in selecting materials and activities is to observe rhythm, frequency, intensity and duration of the oral sensorimotor experiences the child is seeking and creating.

Observations of oral motor preferences coupled with previously obtained information from a thorough sensory history (which includes food preferences and oral self regulatory strategies) will create the menu for therapeutic opportunities and growth. A wide variety of activities and materials should be available. Oral motor skills are naturally complex and the variations of combinations of skills endless. For this reason children normally only spend a short amount of time on each activity, be it a whistle, biting and tugging on a piece of tubing, jerky or licorice, chewing gum or sucking on a piece of hard candy. It is the changes and combinations of activities that promote integration and functional oral motor skill as well as provide support to other layers of the model.

Treatment Guidelines

♦ The SSB synchrony must be addressed to both access and activate the synergy for refinement and elaboration.

♦ The SSB synergy may be accessed in order to activate the developmental areas in the outer layers of the model for more efficient performance.

♦ Honor what the child knows. Use it as a guide to plan treatment (set goals and objectives) and work from strength.

Excerpts from: *MORE: Integrating the Mouth with Sensory and Postural Functions*, 1995. PDP Press, Inc. Printed with permission.

Therapeutic Listening™ Program Follow Up Form

Client's Name:_____Date: _____

Date Program Implemented:_____

Current Prescribed Program: _____

Name of Person Contacting Client: _____

1. What is the current total listening time? _____

    How consistent has this been? _____

    How has the client responded in terms of following the program? _____

    _____

    _____

2. Please describe any changes in emotional tone (i.e. more excited, more irritable, more ani-
    mated) _____

    _____

    _____

3. Please describe any changes in arousal (i.e. general energy level, sleep/wake patterns, transi-
    tions) _____

    _____

    _____

4. Please describe any changes in motor skill (i.e. participation in activity, gross motor coordina-
    tion, handwriting)_____

    _____

    _____

5. Please describe any changes in self care routines (i.e. dressing, toileting, eating, follow through
    with directions, level of independence) _____

    _____

    _____

6. Please describe any changes in social behavior (i.e. language, interactions with peers and others, interactions with family) _____

_____

_____

_____

7. Anything else? _____

_____

_____

Modifications Recommended for Therapeutic Listening Program:
(to be completed by therapist if there are any concerns or questions expressed by family/client; otherwise, continue with initially prescribed Therapeutic Listening progression)

1. Disc # 1: _____ Time: _____

2. Disc # 2 _____ Time: _____

3. Disc # 3 _____ Time: _____

Comments

Month: _____

Level of Change Made:
0 = No Change
1 +/- = Little Change

Name: _____

Areas of Need / Behaviors:

A. Touch
B. Attention
C. Play
D. Activity
E. Communication
F. Auditory Sensitivity

G. Motor Skills
H. Sleep
I. Emotional/Behavioral
J. Self-cares
K. Eating habits
L. Social Skills

CD: 1) _____
2) _____

_____ Minutes
_____ Times\Day

Sun	Mon	Tue	Wed	Thu	Fri	Sat

May be reproduced for home and clinic use *Listening with the Whole Body*

THERAPEUTIC LISTENING™ HOME PROGRAM

Client:_____Therapist:_____ Date: _____

CD#1 _____ CD#2 _____

Offer the following sensory diet items for the listener to choose from:

Deep pressure touch is firm touch like massage.
Proprioception is the sensation of joints and muscles. These joint senses give information about the movement, location and force exerted on joints and muscles.
Heavy work is a kind of proprioception and includes anything that makes muscles work against resistance.

This includes whole body action and is best described as push, pull, lift, play, move! Use of hands, as in fidgeting with toys is also heavy work.
Oral such as chewing, sucking, blowing. Helps to focus and organize. Use in meals, snacks and at play. This is like heavy work for the mouth.
Movement such as swinging, rocking, jumping, tumbling, etc. are particularly powerful especially when done in specific positions. Rhythmic movement is also very calming in contrast to fast changeable movement.

MINUTES FOR:

DAY	CD#1	CD#2	
			____Emotions ____Sleep/Wake ____Eating/Thirst ____Bowel/Bladder ____Behavior **additional notes:**
			____Emotions ____Sleep/Wake ____Eating/Thirst ____Bowel/Bladder ____Behavior **additional notes:**
			____Emotions ____Sleep/Wake ____Eating/Thirst ____Bowel/Bladder ____Behavior **additional notes:**
			____Emotions ____Sleep/Wake ____Eating/Thirst ____Bowel/Bladder ____Behavior **additional notes:**
			____Emotions ____Sleep/Wake ____Eating/Thirst ____Bowel/Bladder ____Behavior **additional notes:**
			____Emotions ____Sleep/Wake ____Eating/Thirst ____Bowel/Bladder ____Behavior **additional notes:**
			____Emotions ____Sleep/Wake ____Eating/Thirst ____Bowel/Bladder ____Behavior **additional notes:**

Initially you may notice an increase in sensitivity and emotionality. This is in response to the high intensity of sensory input and is only temporary. Initially, while listening, it would be helpful to offer some of the options your therapist checked at the top of the page. This will assist in keeping the nervous system at an optimal level of organization.

You may also notice an increase in thirst or hunger throughout the day during the listening program. If you notice an increase in emotionality or any other behaviors which are uncontrollable, stop the program and contact one of our occupational therapists.

SPECIAL INSTRUCTIONS: _____

Sheila M. Frick, with contributions from Children's Therapy Clinic, 1997.

HOME PROGRAM
EASE DISC/ MODULATED MUSIC

Name : _____ **Start Date:** _____

Follow-Up Appointment: _____ **Home Phone:** _____

General Information:

The headphones have a right and left ear designated. The headphone with the wire goes on the left ear. It is important to have the headphones on correctly because of the way the music is recorded. The headphones recommended are engineered to the same quality at which the discs are recorded. Headphones utilized should have an impedance of 150 Ohms and a sensitivity range to 22,000 Hz. Using a lesser headphone will not support the same potential outcomes from a Therapeutic Listening program.

Your CD player should have the following features: a random play feature and the ability to turn off the bass boost feature (if your player has a bass booster). Also, when you listen to the CD player over headphones, the volume should be equal in each headphone throughout the full range of possible volumes. Additionally, when listening through headphones, no background noises (i.e. hisses, pops, static) should be noticeable.

Listening should be done at a comfortable volume. This may mean that at times the ears have to reach for the sound due to the way the CDs are recorded. The volume is too high if the listener seems to be speaking in a loud voice during conversation. The music should never be played at a loud volume. Music played at loud volumes or with heavy bass should NEVER be listened to over headphones.

Each time before beginning the listening, hit the random play feature on the CD. This is so each listening session will be a little different. If the CD player does not have a random play feature, start the CD on the track where it left off during the previous listening session.

You may wish to purchase a Tune Belt if your child will be using a portable CD player. The Tune Belt allows for greater mobility while listening.

Activities discouraged while listening: TV, video games, computer use, or anything that seems to make the listener unavailable (i.e. lining up toys). Anything else, including eating and drinking, is okay. Movement and sensorimotor activities may be helpful if initiated by the listener.

Listening Program:

1. Listen to _____ for _____ minutes _____times a day.
   Each session should be separated by 3 hours.
2. Strategies to support your child during listening might include:

If you have any questions or if any uncharacteristic behaviors occur, please call. _____

THERAPEUTIC LISTENING™ HOME PROGRAM

Name : _____ **Start Date:** _____

Follow-Up Appointment: _____ **Home Phone:** _____

General Information:

The headphones have a right and left ear designated. The headphone with the wire goes on the left ear. It is important to have the headphones on correctly because of the way the music is recorded. The headphones recommended are engineered to the same quality at which the discs are recorded. Headphones utilized should have an impedance of 150 Ohms and a sensitivity range to 22,000 Hz. Using a lesser headphone will not support the same potential outcomes from a Therapeutic Listening program.

Your CD player should have the following features: a random play feature; the ability to turn off the bass boost feature (if your player has a bass booster). Additionally, when you listen to the CD player over headphones, the volume should be equal in each headphone throughout the full range of possible volumes. Also, when listening through headphones, no background noises (i.e. hisses, pops, static) should be noticeable.

Listening should be done at a comfortable volume. This may mean that at times the ears have to reach for the sound due to the way the CDs are recorded. The volume is too high if the listener seems to be speaking in a loud voice during conversation. The music should never be played at a loud volume. Music played at loud volumes or with heavy bass should NEVER be listened to over headphones.

Each time before beginning the listening, hit the random play feature on the CD. This is so each listening session will be a little different. If the CD player does not have a random play feature, start the CD on the track where it left off during the previous listening session.

You may wish to purchase a Tune Belt if your child will be using a portable CD player. The Tune Belt allows for greater mobility while listening.

Activities discouraged while listening: TV, video games, computer use, or anything that seems to make the listener unavailable (i.e. lining up toys). Anything else, including eating and drinking, is okay. Movement and sensorimotor activities may be helpful if initiated by the listener.

Listening Program:

1. Listen to _____ for _____ minutes _____ times a day. Increase by _____ minutes every _____ day if no intense behavioral or emotional reactions occur.
2. Use the random play feature during listening sessions so that each listening session is varied.
3. If increased emotionality or uncomfortable, uncharacteristic behaviors are present, stop for a day and consult with us.
4. Listen in the morning or early afternoon unless another time is specified by your therapist.
5. Strategies to support your child during listening might include:

If you have any questions or if any uncharacteristic behaviors occur, please call _____

OCCUPATIONAL THERAPY REFERRAL QUESTIONNAIRE

Date: **General Information**

Child's Name: _____   Date of Birth:_____

Parents/Guardians: _____

Address: _____   Home Phone_____

_____

Father's Place of Employment: _____   Work Phone_____

Mother's Place of Employment: _____   Work Phone _____

Health Insurance Company:_____   Policy Number: _____

Who referred child for occupational therapy services?_____

_____

Developmental and Medical History

1. Please describe your child's birth history. List any complications during pregnancy, birth, or infancy. _____

    _____

    _____

2. Please give the approximate ages that your child accomplished major developmental milestones. Please include sitting independently, crawling, walking, reaching, talking, etc.

    _____

    _____

    _____

3. Please describe any developmental challenges your child has faced or continues to face.

    _____

    _____

    _____

Please use the following scale to describe your child's behavior.
1 - Never or rarely exhibits this behavior
2 - Occasionally exhibits this behavior
3 - Exhibits this behavior as much as is typical for a child of this age
4 - Exhibits this behavior somewhat more often than expected
5 - Very frequently exhibits this behavior

4.	Diarrhea	1	2	3	4	5
5.	Stomachache	1	2	3	4	5
6.	Vomiting	1	2	3	4	5
7.	Headache	1	2	3	4	5
8.	Constipation	1	2	3	4	5
9.	Earache	1	2	3	4	5

10. Does your child have a history of ear infections? If yes, please describe the frequency of occurrence and how the ear infections have been medically treated. _____

_____

_____

11. Does your child have any allergies? If yes, please list what your child is allergic to, how these allergies are medically managed and any behaviors your child exhibits that you think are related either to the allergies or the allergy medications. _____

_____

_____

12. Does your child currently take any medications? If yes, please list the medications, dosages and for what condition the medication is taken. Also, please list any behaviors your child exhibits that you believe might be attributed to the medication. _____

_____

_____

Check any of the following with whom you have had contact concerning your child. (Give name and address)

[ ] Psychologist   [ ] Physical Therapist   [ ] Speech Therapist   [ ] Neurologist
    [ ] Resource of Special Teacher

School History

What is your child's current grade? _____
What school does your child attend at this time? _____

_____

Teacher's Name:_____

Has your child had any formal evaluations/testing? If so, what and when? _____

_____

_____

Behavioral/Emotional Components

Please use the following scale to describe your child's behavior.
1 - Never or rarely exhibits this behavior
2 - Occasionally exhibits this behavior
3 - Exhibits this behavior as much as is typical for a child of this age
4 - Exhibits this behavior somewhat more often than expected
5 - Very frequently exhibits this behavior

1.	Compliant	1	2	3	4	5
2.	Displays affection toward others	1	2	3	4	5
3.	Displays aggression toward self	1	2	3	4	5
4.	Displays aggression toward others	1	2	3	4	5
5.	Irritable	1	2	3	4	5
6.	Cries easily	1	2	3	4	5
7.	Seems happy	1	2	3	4	5
8.	Seems immature for age	1	2	3	4	5
9.	Displays rapid mood swings	1	2	3	4	5
10.	Seems independent	1	2	3	4	5
11.	Seems dependent	1	2	3	4	5
12.	"Baby talks"	1	2	3	4	5
13.	Seems to need a lot of comfort and nurturing	1	2	3	4	5
14.	Seems impulsive	1	2	3	4	5

Communication

Please use the following scale to describe your child's behavior.
1 - Never or rarely exhibits this behavior
2 - Occasionally exhibits this behavior
3 - Exhibits this behavior as much as is typical for a child of this age
4 - Exhibits this behavior somewhat more often than expected
5 - Very frequently exhibits this behavior

1.	Initiates eye contact when greeting someone	1	2	3	4	5
2.	Initiates eye contact when requesting information	1	2	3	4	5
3.	Sustains eye contact	1	2	3	4	5
4.	Takes turns	1	2	3	4	5
5.	Interacts with peers	1	2	3	4	5
6.	Interacts with adults	1	2	3	4	5
7.	Participates in conversations	1	2	3	4	5
8.	Responds to verbal information in a timely manner (little lag in response time)	1	2	3	4	5

9. If your child is nonverbal, please describe the frequency and types of vocalizations your child uses. _____

_____

_____

10. If your child is nonverbal, please describe how your child communicates and give examples.

_____

_____

_____

11. If your child is verbal, please describe your child's verbal abilities (i.e. vocabulary, ability to stay on topic, etc.) _____

_____

_____

Self-Care/Daily Routines

1. Please describe a typical mealtime with your child. Include where, what and how your child eats, your child's typical appetite, the number of meals and snacks your child has each day, your child's behavior during mealtimes, etc.

_____

_____

_____

2. Please describe how your child typically gets dressed. Include the types of clothing your child wears, how independent your child is with his/her clothing, how long it takes your child to dress, your child's behavior during dressing, etc. _____

_____

_____

3. Please describe a typical bath time for your child. Include your child's level of independence in bathing, your child's like or dislike for bath time, your child's behavior during bath time, etc. _____

_____

_____

4. Please describe your child's behavior and level of independence for each of the following tasks:

Teeth brushing _____

_____

_____

Hair brushing _____

_____

_____

Washing hands and face _____

_____

_____

5. Please describe your child's toileting skills. Include level of independence, frequency of occurrences of bed wetting, frequency of occurrences of daytime bowel and bladder accidents, awareness of toileting needs, etc. _____

_____

_____

6. Please describe how your child makes transitions between people or environments. Include level of independence during transitions, need for transitional objects, need for advance preparation about schedule changes, etc. _____

_____

_____

7. If applicable, please describe how your child completes homework. Include level of independence, need for breaks, need for external supports (food, music, etc.), the amount of time typically needed, etc. _____

_____

_____

8. Please describe your child's ability to independently keep track of personal belongings.

_____

_____

_____

9. Please describe your child's ability to independently organize personal belongings (homework, bedroom, desk, etc.). _____

_____

_____

10. Please describe your child's typical play skills. Include information about the ages of the people your child chooses to play with, if your child chooses to be a leader, a follower, or a loner, how many people your child is comfortable playing with at once, whether your child prefers a few close friends or a lot of acquaintances, etc. _____

_____

_____

_____

Arousal/Attention/Self-Regulation

Please use the following scale to describe your child's behavior.
1 - Never or rarely exhibits this behavior
2 - Occasionally exhibits this behavior
3 - Exhibits this behavior as much as is typical for a child of this age
4 - Exhibits this behavior somewhat more often than expected
5 - Very frequently exhibits this behavior

1.	Is an early morning riser	1	2	3	4	5
2.	Awakens during the night	1	2	3	4	5
3.	Has difficulty falling asleep	1	2	3	4	5
4.	Is irritable upon awakening	1	2	3	4	5
5.	Wets bed	1	2	3	4	5
6.	Attends to toys	1	2	3	4	5
7.	Attends at school	1	2	3	4	5
8.	Attends in new environments	1	2	3	4	5
9.	Able to independently sustain attention	1	2	3	4	5
10.	Independently explores	1	2	3	4	5

11. Please describe the following (include behaviors your child exhibits that you think are significant, any tricks you use to help your child during these times, etc):

a typical bed time routine _____

_____

_____

a typical night's sleep _____

_____

_____

a typical wake-up routine _____

_____

_____

12. Does your child seem irritable at predictable times of the day? If yes, please describe the times of the day when your child seems irritable and the events that seem likely to trigger irritability. _____

_____

_____

13. Does your child seem happier or more cooperative at predictable times of the day? If yes, please describe the times of the day when your child seems happiest and most cooperative and the events that seem likely to precede these behaviors. _____

_____

_____

14. Please describe how your child approaches and explores a new environment.

_____

_____

_____

15. Please describe any strategies your child uses to help himself/herself sustain focused attention.

_____

_____

_____

Sensory Components

1. Please describe your child's sensitivity to touch. Include information about your child's behavior regarding being touched, any clothing preferences your child might have, how your child uses touch to explore, etc. _____

_____

_____

2. Please describe your child's sensitivity to movement. Include information about the types of movement your child likes and dislikes, the frequency with which your child seems to seek movement, your child's behavior regarding being moved or lifted off the ground, etc.

_____

_____

_____

3. Please describe your child's sensitivity to sound. Include any types of sounds your child particularly enjoys or particularly dislikes, your child's ability to filter out irrelevant sounds, your child's behavior regarding loud sounds, etc. _____

_____

_____

_____

4. Please describe your child's visual attention. Include information about sensitivity to light, ability to attend to relevant visual information, ability to sustain visual attention, what typically engages your child's visual attention, etc. _____

_____

_____

_____

Balance/Body Awareness/Praxis

Please use the following scale to describe your child's behavior.
1 - Never or rarely exhibits this behavior
2 - Occasionally exhibits this behavior
3 - Exhibits this behavior as much as is typical for a child of this age
4 - Exhibits this behavior somewhat more often than expected
5 - Very frequently exhibits this behavior

1.	Initiates new activities	1	2	3	4	5
2.	Understands how to play with new/novel toys	1	2	3	4	5
3.	Plays with same toy in a variety of ways	1	2	3	4	5
4.	Able to perform sequential tasks	1	2	3	4	5
5.	Jumps	1	2	3	4	5
6.	Plays on playground equipment (slides, jungle gym, monkey bars, etc.)	1	2	3	4	5
7.	Swings	1	2	3	4	5
8.	Enjoys roughhouse type play	1	2	3	4	5
9.	Takes risks	1	2	3	4	5
10.	Seems aware of safety concerns	1	2	3	4	5

11. Does your child ride a bicycle? If so, please describe what type of bike your child rides, how much assistance your child needs to get on and off the bike and ride the bike, how frequently your child rides his/her bike, etc. _____

_____

_____

12. Please describe how your child ascends and descends stairs.

_____

_____

_____

13. In your own words, describe your child's general level of motor coordination. Include types of motor experiences your child enjoys, your child's independence in initiating motor experiences, how much assistance and supervision your child needs during motor play, etc.

_____

_____

_____

14. In your own words, please describe your child's balance skills.

_____

_____

_____

Parental Concerns

1. What do you see as your child's strengths? _____

_____

_____

_____

2. What are your concerns about your child? _____

_____

_____

3. What have you been told by doctors, teachers and/or others about your child's abilities and needs? _____

_____

_____

4. What do you hope will be gained by having your child seen at this clinic?

_____

_____

Revised 8/98. From Susan Buck, MS, OTR/L, Colleen Hacker, MS, OTR/L and Dawn Schinaman, OTR/L (Developmental Therapy Associates, Inc). - 12/94
Adapted from information from Sheila Frick, OTR (Therapeutic Resources, Madison, WI)

Clinical Reasoning for Selection of Music

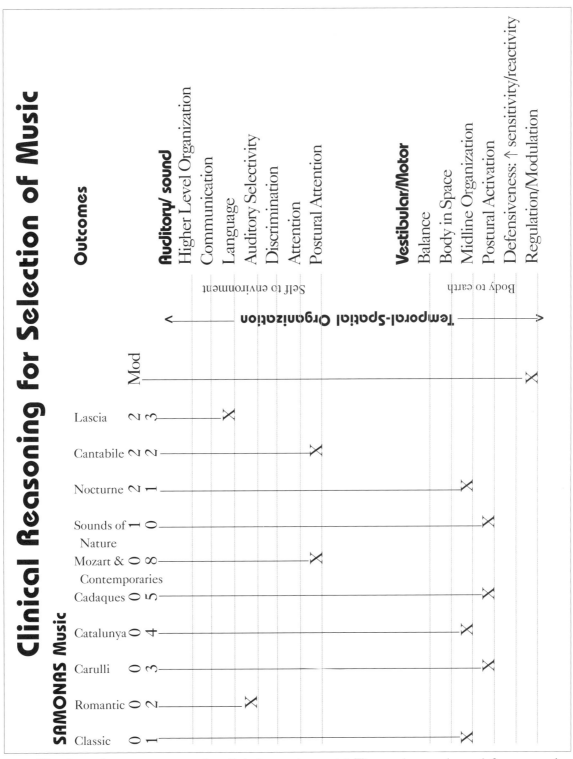

The above chart represents another clinical reasoning model. The numbers on the top left correspond to music selections. The lines extending from each number correlate to the level of function or skill where each CD might have an impact.

CD selection should occur on the basis of which behaviors are being targeted. Functions or other skills related to the vestibular portion of the system should be addressed prior to functions or skills related to the auditory portion of the system. When vestibular or body-related issues are addressed first, other more refined skills may be uncovered. Choose level of intensity of spectral activation (CQ, HS, SE, ST) according to the individual's need for detailed information for finer discrimination.

References/Suggested Readings

Assagioli, R. (1991). Music: Cause of disease and healing agent. In D. Campbell (Ed.), *Music: physician for times to come* (97-108). Wheaton, IL: The Theosophical Publishing House.

Ayres, A. J. (1972). *Sensory integration and learning disorders.* Los Angeles: Western Psychological Services.

Ayres, A. J. (1979). *Sensory integration and the child.* Los Angeles: Western Psychological Services.

Backus, J. (1977). *The acoustical foundations of music.* New York: W.W. Norton & Co.

Beery, K. E., Buktenica, N. A. (1997). *Developmental test of visual motor integration.* Parsippany, NJ: Modern Curriculum Press, Simon & Schuster.

Brewer, C. & Campbell, D. G. (1991). *Rhythms of learning.* Tucson, AZ: Zephyr Press, Inc.

Campbell, D. (2000). *The Mozart effect for children: Awakening your child's mind, health and creativity with music.* New York: Harper Collins Publishers, Inc.

Cogan, R. & Escot, R. (1976). *Sonic design: The nature of sound and music.* Englewood Cliffs, NJ: Prentice-Hall.

Dunn, W. (1999). *The sensory profile.* Austin, TX: The Psychological Corporation.

Erickson, R. (1975). *Sound Structure in Music.* Berkeley, CA: University of California Press.

Folio, M. R., & Fewell, R. R. (1983). *Peabody developmental motor scales.* Allen, TX: DLM Teaching Resources.

Gardner, M. (1985). *Test of auditory perceptual skills (TAPS).* San Francisco, CA: Children's Hospital.

Gardner, K. (1990). *Sounding the Inner Landscape: Music as Medicine.* Stonington, ME: Caduceus Publications.

Goldman, R., Fristoe, M. & Woodcock, R. (1970). *Goldman-Fristoe test of auditory discrimination.* Circle Pines, MN: American Guidance Service.

Harris, D. B. (1963). *Goodenough-Harris drawing test.* San Antonio: Pyschological Corporation, Harcourt Brace & Company.

Jourdain, R. (1997). *Music, the brain and ecstacy: How music captures our imagination.* New York: Avon Books.

Keith, R. W. (2000). *The test for auditory processing disorders in Children (SCAN-C).* Austin, TX: The Psychological Corporation.
(2000). *The test for auditory processing disorders in adolescents and adults (SCAN-A).* Austin, TX: The Psychological Corporation.

Kimball, J. G. (1993). Sensory integrative frame of reference. In Kramer, P. & Hinojosa, J. (Eds.) *Frames of reference for pediatric occupational therapy.* Baltimore, MD: Williams & Wilkins.

Levarie, S. & Levy, E. (1980). *Tone: A study in musical acoustics.* Kent, OH: Kent State University Press.

Lindamood, P. (1997). *Lindamood auditory conceptualization.* Austin, TX: PRO-ED, Inc.

Madaule, P. (1998, Spring). Listening training and music education. *Early Childhood Connections: Journal of Music- and Movement-Based Learning, 4* (2), 34-41.

Madaule, P. (1997, Spring). Music: An invitation to listening, language and learning. *Early childhood Connections: Journal of Music- and Movement-Based Learning, 3* (2).

Miller, L. J., Reisman, J. E., McIntosh, D. N., & Simon, J. (2001). An ecological model of sensory modulation: Performance of children with fragile X syndrome, autistic disorder, attention-deficit/hyperactivity disorder, and sensory modulation dysfunction. In Roley, S., Blanche, E. & Schaaf, R. (Eds.), *Understanding the Nature of Sensory integration with diverse populations* (pp. 57-82). San Antonio, TX: Therapy Skill Builders, A Harcourt Health Sciences Company.

Morris, S. E. (1991). Facilitation of learning. Reprinted with permission from M. B. Langley and L. J. Lombardino. *Neurodevelopmental strategies for managing communication disorders in children with severe motor dysfunction* Austin, TX: Pro-ed.

Morris, S. (1992). *The normal acquisition of oral feeding skills. Implications for assessment and treatment.* New York: Therapeutic Media.

Oetter, P., Richter, E. & Frick, S. (1995). *MORE: Integrating the mouth with sensory and postural functions, 2nd Edition.* Hugo, MN: PDP Press, Inc.

Oetter, P. (1986). Assessment: The child with attention deficit disorder. *Sensory Integration Special Interest Section Newsletter,* 9 (1), 6-7. Rockville, MD. American Occupational Therapy Association.

Reisman, J. (1999). *Minnesota handwriting test user's manual.* San Antonio: The Psychological Corporation.

Richter, E., Montgomery, P. (1989). *The sensorimotor performance analysis.* Hugo, MN: PDP Press, Inc.

Rimland, B., Edelson, S. (1999). *Autism treatment evaluation checklist (ATEC).* Retrieved April 1, 2002, from http://www.autism.com/ari

Shaw, G. L. (2000). *Keeping Mozart in mind.* San Diego, CA: Academic Press.

Stackhouse, T. & Wilbarger, J. (1998). *Occupational therapy perspectives of sensory modulation disorders.* Retrieved April 2, 2002, from http://www.SINet.org

Steinbach, I. (1999). *SAMONAS sound therapy handbook.* Kellinghusen, Germany: Techau Verlag.

Steinbach, I. (2000). http://www.samonas.com

Tame, D. (1984). *The secret power of music.* New York: Destiny Books.

Thaut, M., Schleiffers, S., Davis, W. (1991). Analysis of EMG activity in biceps and triceps muscle in an upper extremity gross motor task under the influence of auditory rhythm. *Journal of Music Therapy,* 28, 64-88.

White, H. E. & H. D. (1980). *Physics and music: The science of musical sound.* Philadelphia, PA: Saunders College.

Wigram, T. & DiLeo, C. (1997). *Music vibration.* Cherry Hill, NJ: Jeffrey Books.

Wilbarger, J. L. (1998). The emerging concept of sensory modulation disorders. *Sensory Integration Special Interest Section Newsletter,* 21 (3), 3-4. Bethesda, MD: AOTA.

Wilbarger, P. (1984). Planning an adequate sensory diet: Application of sensory processing theory during the first year of life. *Zero to Three: National Center for Clinical Infant Programs, V* (1).

Wilbarger, P. & Wilbarger, J. L. (1991). *Sensory defensiveness in children aged 2-12: An intervention guide for parents and other caretakers.* Santa Barbara, CA: Avanti Educational Programs.

Wilbarger, P. & Wilbarger, J. L. (2001). *Sensory defensiveness: A comprehensive treatment approach.* Workshop handouts. Santa Barbara, CA: Avanti Education Programs.

Clinical Reasoning and Documented Outcomes

4

Contents

Name: John
Age: 8.0 years

This child exhibits some characteristics of a mild sensory modulation dysfunction & listening difficulties. His program typifies an initial listening protocol.

Referral Information

John was referred for an occupational therapy assessment due to questions regarding his sensory processing. Concerns had arisen at school regarding the possibility of attention deficit disorder because he demonstrates restless and fidgety behavior. He works with a private psychologist who believes John has a mild anxiety disorder but rates very low for attention deficit disorder. John is challenged at school to adhere to the rules and regulations of a typical classroom environment. His parents are concerned that John's self-esteem may be affected by his difficulty performing up to classroom expectations.

John was the product of induced labor. He was jaundiced at birth and remained under bilirubin lights for almost a week, but otherwise was a healthy infant; all early motor and language milestones were accomplished within expected intervals. John does, however, have a history of persistent middle ear infections. He has had his adenoids removed and has had pressure equalizing (PE) tubes placed in his ears twice. John also seems to have stomachaches and constipation more often than typical. Lately, the question has arisen as to whether John's frequent stomachaches are related to anxiety about school.

Currently John attends second grade. He receives no support services through the public schools. John has been evaluated by a child psychiatrist and has received ongoing private counseling services for the past eighteen months.

John's parents perceive his strength to be his personality, describing him as having a lot of character. They are most concerned about his self-esteem and lack of confidence. They worry that school may be creating increased anxiety for him by expecting a higher level of performance than he can consistently muster. John and his family have come to Therapeutic Resources seeking information, resources and intervention that might help alleviate some of his struggles. They are seeking tools that could be used at home, as well as translated to a school environment, so that John may be comfortable there.

Assessment/Observations

Prior to any clinical assessment of John's behavior and motor skills, the Developmental Test of Visual-Motor Integration (VMI), the Test for Auditory Processing Disorders in Children (SCAN-C) and the screening for the Interactive Metronome® (IM) were administered, with the following results:

John's scores on the VMI were all at or above expected age performance. He had no difficulty with any of these tasks. His score on the Visual-Motor Integration subtest, while solidly average, was his lowest relative score.

John was left-handed. He held his pencil in an appropriate tripod grasp. No notable motor challenges were observed that would interfere with John's ability to competently and efficiently complete visual-motor activities within an educational environment.

John achieved average or above average scores on the subtests of the SCAN-C with the exception of his performance on the Filtered Words subtest. As the auditory information presented became more complex, John became a little more restless and fidgety in his chair. He seemed to become less confident in his responses as the testing progressed. Functionally, John's listening perception may be weighted more toward the focusing aspect of listening than the monitoring aspect. A dynamic balance between the two functions is what is desired. John may be 'tuned in' to the details of his environment more often than is helpful. Therefore, sounds like pencils scratching on paper and fans blowing may catch his attention and distract him from task. Most auditory elements in the environment seem brought to the foreground; therefore, John perceives everything as if it were important and can't select what is the most salient or relevant information.

John also demonstrated discrepancy between his left and right ears for listening. His right ear performance was consistently higher than his left ear.

John's middle ear mechanism does not appear to be functioning with the expected level of flexibility. It may be difficult for him to create an appropriate balance between auditory foreground and background, so focusing on specific auditory information (i.e. the teacher's voice) with accuracy may be challenging. He may become over stimulated in 'busy' auditory environments and simply tune out. He may also attempt to utilize sensorimotor strategies (such as movement or chewing) to help focus his attention. However, these strategies seem to create controversy as to whether John is actually able to attend within a classroom setting.

Interactive Metronome®

The Interactive Metronome®, a computerized program that assesses rhythmic motor control, was used with John. IM measures the milliseconds (ms.) it takes for an individual to respond to a rhythmic target stimulus. The individual responds to the target stimulus through a variety of motor patterns (clapping hands, tapping

toes, tapping heels, etc.). John's performance ranged from 52 ms. to 264 ms. An average performance for a child of John's age would be a response within 50-90 ms. John's performance would be considered in the 'at risk' range, with probable sequencing, timing and planning problems.

General Observations

During the initial standardized portion of the testing, John was attentive and focused. As the testing progressed, John became restless and slightly fidgety, specifically, shuffling and swinging his feet under his chair. Several times, he asked if he were almost finished. However, though John was slightly restless, at no time did his extra movement interfere with his ability to complete tasks. He was able to work diligently for a period of 60 minutes with minimal redirection or external support.

The testing situation represented 'ideal' conditions for John and he may have been able to demonstrate his best performance. He had 1:1 adult attention, a relatively quiet, distraction-free environment and novelty of circumstance. However, 60 minutes is a long period of time in which to sustain attention to task for any child. Clinical experience suggests that John needs sensorimotor support in order to adequately sustain attention over time, but he is able to generate strategies through movement in his chair and input to his mouth (chewing on objects) that help him with this endeavor. The question becomes how to incorporate John's needs for sensorimotor strategies to sustain an optimal arousal state into actions that are permissible within his classroom environment.

Instructional note #1: *Interpreting information binaurally (from both ears) may be challenging in instances where there is a listening discrepancy in performance between the two ears. In turn, difficulty interpreting information binaurally may lead to spatial and perceptual confusion. This spatial and directional confusion may lead to behaviors that look like distractibility, inattentiveness and a restlessness in the environment.*

Instructional note #2: *The middle ear mechanism (specifically, the stapedius muscle) relaxes and contracts to monitor the ambient environment and focus in on specific information. The monitoring function allows one to notice and then disregard all of the background sounds in an environment; the focusing function allows one to tune in to the most pertinent or salient auditory information present.*

John's performance demonstrates how very competent and capable he is. The challenges that he faces in daily life should then be considered reflective of his inability to consistently access his highest level of performance. This inconsistency may be a sign of poor or inefficient integration and organization of information received through his senses.

> *Instructional Note #3: Children's sensory needs are often much more intense than the needs of adults. They may have difficulty remaining in their seats, remaining still when they are in their seats, modulating the volume of their voices, or keeping their body parts to themselves. However, if these behaviors are viewed as needs, or requirements for the children's sensory diets, rather than as problems or difficulties, the methods of handling these behaviors is altered.*

Interpretation

John's performance during this assessment suggests challenges in two significant areas. First, John appears to be significantly challenged in the perceptual process of listening. While his 'hearing' seems fine, his ability to filter relevant from irrelevant information is effected. He seems to perceive all sounds as if they are important. Thus, in a classroom, it might be challenging for John to direct attention. The chairs scraping on the floor, the door closing down the hall, or the teacher's voice are all given equal importance perceptually. Therefore, when John seems not to be listening, he is listening to everything as if it is equally important. Because everything is given equal value, he may lose some of the information, such as part of the instructions provided by the teacher.

Secondly, John seems to have mild difficulties regulating his own level of arousal. His need to move in his seat and to chew on objects signal that John is having some difficulty modulating his level of arousal. Often the very behaviors that seem to suggest inattention are the behaviors that help sustain attention. As adults, we have all incorporated behaviors, our personal sensory diets, into our lives that help us to remain attentive. These behaviors are so subtle and so much a part of us that often we do not realize that we are doing them, such as chewing on a pencil, drumming fingers, wiggling toes, tapping feet, or shifting in a chair.

Rather than viewing John's motor restlessness as a deterrent, he should be given permis-

sion to continue with this behavior. In this way, he is regulating his state of attention and arousal to the best of his ability. What becomes essential in a classroom environment is to find ways to address John's sensory needs in a manner that does not interfere with the learning environment for other students.

Plan

Listening Program
☊ Initiate use of a Therapeutic Listening program with EASe Disc 1 to help address issues regarding auditory discrimination and auditory sensitivity. Listening time should be 2X daily for 30 minute listening sessions. A minimum of 3 hours should separate listening times.

Concurrent Treatment Suggestions

✌ John is a good candidate for the Interactive Metronome. Timing of this intervention should occur during the summer months when John has fewer commitments.

✌ It will be important to address John's challenges with auditory information in the classroom. He should be seated near the teacher but also in a place where he is not in a highly trafficked area or where he is seated next to something that makes continual noise (such as a heater).

✌ Auditory instructions should be paired with visual instructions.

✌ A quiet corner for completing work should be an option for John as well as for other children in the classroom, such as a study carrel in the back of the classroom, seated facing away from the general traffic of the class.

✌ Because movement seems to be organizing for John, it will be important that opportunities for movement be provided through his day, especially if movement while he is in his seat will be discouraged. Are there other ways in which to build physical activity into John's day? Could he be the class lifter and carrier, moving books around, emptying garbage cans or other created tasks that would involve use of his muscles within the context of a functional activity?

✎   Implementation of an appropriate sensory diet for John across all environments will be important. See appendix: 'Sensory Diet', p. 3-69).

Name: Annie
Age: 6.7 years

Initiating a listening program
with a child diagnosed with
dyslexia and who is demonstrating
mild to moderate sensory
processing problems

Referral Information

Annie was referred for an occupational therapy assessment for questions regarding her sensory processing. She has been diagnosed as dyslexic. One of the characteristics of Annie's dyslexia is that the symbols 'dance around' on a page when she attempts to read. The possibility of sensory integration dysfunction has also been raised, particularly regarding her general ability to regulate. She seems sensitive to touch and to certain sounds, loves swinging and moves a lot but gets carsick and, visually, can over focus on a computer but have difficulty focusing on printed material in a book. Annie also has difficulty regulating her sleep/wake cycles. It takes her approximately an hour to fall asleep at night. She sleeps solidly for 9 hours but has to be awakened by a parent or she would sleep for 11 hours if left to wake on her own.

Annie was the product of induced labor. She was difficult to nurse and had chronic colic from 2 weeks to 4 months of age. All language and motor milestones were accomplished within expected intervals. Though she crawled at 8 months, she did not linger at this stage, as she did not like to be on her stomach. She cruised at 9 months and walked independently at 10 months. By the time Annie was one, she no longer napped.

Annie attends first grade. She is enrolled in a gifted and talented program. She has also attended a learning center for correction of dyslexia in which she learned some visualization techniques to aid her thinking and decoding processes.

Annie's parents perceive her strengths to be her sense of humor, her visual ability, her intellectual ability and her warm heart. They are concerned about Annie's ability to perform in school and enjoy learning. They would like to see her feel comfortable a greater percentage of the time. They also have questions about other diagnostic considerations, wondering about how factors such as boredom, possible sleep disorder and possible sensory integration dysfunction might complicate or confound her clinical picture. They've come to Therapeutic Resources seeking information, resources and intervention that might help Annie and alleviate her struggles.

Assessment/Observations

During the initial, standardized portion of the testing, Annie was quite subdued. She demonstrated adequate concentration and was able to complete all tasks efficiently and without great effort. She did occasionally ask for directions to be repeated. In general, the tasks presented did not challenge Annie's inherent brightness. As such, she seemed well able to compensate for higher level challenges. However, as the context itself grew more challenging, Annie's subtle difficulties became more apparent.

Annie's mother related that her overall demeanor was not typical. She described Annie as typically being a very active, energetic child, in constant motion and with some difficulty focusing and concentrating. It is certainly not unusual for any child to be on 'best behavior' in a novel environment with novel adults. Annie's performance on standardized assessment instruments may be reflective of her peak effort. Had testing proceeded much longer, Annie may not have been able to sustain this level of effort and a more typical performance might have been elicited. However, Annie's performance does demonstrate how very competent and capable she is. The challenges she faces in daily life should then be considered reflective of her inability to consistently access her highest level of performance. This inconsistency may be a sign of poor or inefficient integration and organization of information received through her senses.

Prior to any clinical assessment of Annie's behavior and motor skills, the Developmental Test of Visual-Motor Integration (VMI), the Test for Auditory Processing Disorders in Children (SCAN-C) and the screening for the Interactive Metronome were administered, with the following results:

Annie's scores on the VMI were all at or above expected age performance. She had no difficulty with any of these tasks. For a child of Annie's intelligence, the level of challenge on these tasks was relatively low and suspected difficulties with visual-motor integration may have been masked by Annie's ability to cognitively compensate. Her score on the Motor Coordination subtest, while solidly average, was her lowest relative score and it was noted that Annie's handwriting is generally poor. When provided with the degree of structure present on the VMI as well as when under conditions promoting optimal performance, Annie is able to attain average performance; under more ordinary or daily circumstances, Annie seems less able to consistently produce average writing and drawing samples.

Also, when asked to draw a picture of a person, Annie drew a very simple stick figure. Her writing beneath the drawing was characterized by poor spatial organization (upward drift, exaggerated spacing between words, segmentation of letters). With less guidance or external cues to structure her performance, Annie's written products were below age level expectations.

Annie achieved average or above average scores on the subtests of the SCAN-C. As the auditory information presented became more complex, Annie became a little more restless and fidgety in her chair. She seemed to become less confident in her responses as the testing progressed. Functionally, however, the auditory channel appears to be a strong channel for Annie. In fact, Annie's listening perception may be weighted more toward the focusing aspect of listening than the monitoring aspect. A dynamic balance between the two is what is desired.

Additionally, Annie demonstrated discrepancy between her left and right ears for listening. Her right ear performance was consistently higher than her left ear. (Refer to Instructional Note #1, pg 4-4.)

Annie's middle ear mechanism does not appear to be functioning with the expected level of flexibility (refer to instructional note #2, pg. 4-4). It may be difficult for her to create an appropriate balance between auditory foreground and background, thus focusing on specific auditory information (i.e. the teacher's voice) with accuracy may be challenging. Annie may become overstimulated in busy auditory environments and simply tune out.

Interactive Metronome

The Interactive Metronome, a computerized program that assesses rhythmic motor control, was used with Annie (see p. 4-4). An average performance for a child of Annie's age would be a response within 50-90 ms. Annie's performance would be considered to be in the 'at risk' range, with probable sequencing, timing and planning problems.

Due to the short nature of the items presented (i.e. approximately 30 seconds per item), Annie seemed able to concentrate and cognitively compensate for challenges with sequencing and timing. More complex motor patterns had to be presented in order to tap in to her areas of difficulty. For example, Annie was able to clap her hands rhythmically but had difficulty with a task requiring alternate hand and foot movements. Overall, Annie's motor performance lacked fluidity and automaticity.

General Observations

Due to the description of Annie's challenges with her visual system, a few simple visual motor observations were completed. Annie had no post rotary nystagmus following spinning clockwise and counterclockwise. Nystagmus is a reflexive movement of the eyes created by intense stimulation to the vestibular system. It is a reflex that can be used to train smooth visual pursuits and scanning. Additionally, Annie had difficulty with visual fixation at close ranges (6"-18"). While she could fixate on a target at further distances, she moved her head around a lot while trying to get a visual 'lock' at a shorter distance. This would correspond to Annie's experience of the symbols on a page dancing when she is attempting to read. As a compensation for the lack of stability in her visual fixation, she moves her head around to follow the figures that seem to be moving in front of her.

> *Instructional Note #4:* *The visual and auditory systems form two-thirds of a sensorimotor triad. The vestibular system is the remaining element of this triad and can be likened to the tripod of a camera. The vestibular system responds to gravity and plays a large role in balance, mediation of postural tone and overall state regulation and level of arousal. The vestibular sense is the sense against which all other senses are referenced. However, if any component of the vestibular-visual-auditory triad is weak, inefficient, or impaired, the other components are affected as well. It is the manner in which the triad functions and integrates that defines one's perception.*

The longer Annie spent in the clinic, the more her typical behaviors emerged. She sought intense movement experiences, especially combining movement with crashing and jumping. She also moved rapidly from one idea or thought to the next, not sustaining focus or interest in any one activity for long. Though she sought a lot of sensory input, she did not allow herself periods of time in which the information might organize or integrate for her. She didn't seem to have a sense of filling the container. Thus her arousal state subtly wobbles around a midpoint, but she doesn't easily attain or maintain an optimal arousal state. Her need for movement seems to serve two purposes. First, she apparently tries to create a reference point for her body in an environment by stimulating her vestibular system to establish a sense of 'you-are-here.' Second, the vestibular system has myriad connections with the reticular formation that is a major governing influence for determining arousal state and regulation.

Interpretation

Annie seems most reliant on her auditory system; however, her auditory system cannot stand alone. Vision should be laid upon a foundation created by the vestibular and auditory systems. The interaction of these systems is what creates perception. Perception is what gives one an understanding of time and space.

Annie cannot organize in space and time because she does not perceive them in a typical way. Without an understanding of the three-dimensionality of space, Annie cannot efficiently move through it. It is not surprising then, that she chooses to move perpetually, trying to generate enough input to her nervous system to give her the information of where she is in space.

Annie also does not appear to be organized in time. Her lack of motor fluidity in her writing and in her performance on the Interactive Metronome demonstrates this.

Plan

Listening Program

🎧 Initiate use of a Therapeutic Listening program with Mozart for Modulation - Modified to help address issues regarding auditory foreground/background and auditory sensitivity. Listening time should be 2x daily for 30 minute listening sessions. A minimum of 3 hours should separate listening times.

Concurrent Treatment Suggestions

✌ Annie is a good candidate for the Interactive Metronome. Timing of this intervention should occur when the vestibular-auditory-visual triad is more solidly integrated for her.

✌ Annie is also a good candidate for ocular motor treatment. This intervention could precede or correspond with the timing of the IM. Issues to address would be smooth visual pursuits and ability to stabilize visual fixation at near distances.

Name: David
Age: 24 months

Initiating a listening program with a toddler with severe sensory modulation issues compounded by oral, postural and respiratory problems

Referral Information

The primary concern prompting David's referral for an occupational therapy assessment was his challenge with overall state regulation. He has had difficulty gaining weight, beginning primarily with the introduction of solid foods. At the age of two, his weight is more similar to that of an average one year old. He grazes throughout the day and has a very limited repertoire of foods. David also has difficulty sleeping through the night. He typically falls asleep only after a parent rubs his back for approximately 30 minutes. He generally sleeps no longer than four hours waking several times during the night. He is usually up for the day by 4:30 a.m.

David's delivery and early infancy were uneventful. Developmental motor milestones have been accomplished on the late side of typical; David sat independently at 6 months, crawled at 9 months and walked independently at 15 months. His speech development has always been delayed. At 2 years of age, David calls "Mama," "Dada" and "Zsazsa" (the name of his babysitter). He communicates primarily by pointing, pushing or pulling an adult and non-specific vocalizations.

With the exception of the concerns regarding weight gain, David has been a generally physically healthy child. He has no known allergies. He takes a daily multivitamin.

David has been evaluated by Bridges for Families Early Intervention Program and now receives physical therapy and speech therapy services.

From a sensory processing perspective, David demonstrates varying degrees of reactivity or sensitivity to sensory input. As he has gotten older, his sensitivities appear to have lessened. He is slightly sensitive to the tags in clothing. He loves movement and sound, generally the more vigorous the movement or the more stimulating the sound environment, the more satisfying and organizing for David. As a younger child, David was irritable; this is less of an issue now. Still, he appears to be having difficulty sorting, sifting, filtering, integrating, and organizing sensory information for use.

David's parents perceive his strengths to be his sweet, energetic and funny personality. They are most concerned about his disregulated sleep and his poor weight gain. They've come to Therapeutic Resources seeking any information and intervention that might be appropriate for David, especially in the area of regulation.

David's physical therapist evaluated David in December 2000 and has been providing treatment for David regarding postural and respiratory issues. Those issues were not re-assessed during this evaluation.

David entered the clinic without hesitation and readily explored, though he chose to remain in close proximity to his mother and babysitter throughout the time spent. He had no noticeable fears regarding any of the equipment present in the environment and motored his way on and around many obstacles and pieces of equipment. While David readily explored the environment, it took him 15-20 minutes to truly warm up to the therapists and he continued to interact with less familiar adults with slight caution. This is certainly well within the range of typical development.

David indicated his wants and needs through a series of vocalizations and by calling "Mama" and "Zsazsa." He frequently pointed to things in the environment as he called to a familiar adult, indicating his desire to explore something or to ask for assistance.

David lacks jaw stability. He primarily uses the front of his mouth for stability. When food is presented, David chews and suckles the food at the front of his mouth. Three-dimensional chewing patterns and use of the back of jaw for strength and stability have not developed. In an attempt to create more stability, David has developed a pattern of slight retraction through his lips and cheeks. Biomechanically, he is reinforcing less mature patterns of feeding and chewing while recruiting stability through the jaw to compensate for lack of postural stability and organization.

Certainly David's drive toward intensity was apparent while he explored the clinic. He seemed fearless with respect to movement. He was not afraid of heights or of descending from heights. He had varying awareness of safety issues and sometimes stumbled over the edges of things. He seemed to enjoy activities that provided full body impact and created a game of throwing himself on to the mats and pillows.

Because primary referral concerns centered on issues of modulation or regulation, several intervention strategies related to these issues were attempted during David's assessment. The first intervention selected was Therapeutic Listening. Modulated music was chosen for David's listening program.

Nerves that innervate the muscles of the middle ear are neuroanatomically connected to a branch of the vagus nerve. The vagus nerve is connected to many different organs within the body; one of its common roles is that of homeo-

stasis. Through attachment to heart, lungs, digestive organs, bowel, bladder, etc., the vagus nerve has connections to many functions in the body that must maintain rhythmicity in order for equilibrium to be sustained. Regulation of these functions and other rhythmical, cyclical behaviors (such as sleep/wake cycles) is, in part, created by the innervation of the vagus nerve. Thus, using the auditory channel to stimulate these functions often helps create regulation within them as well.

David responded in a mixed fashion to the introduction of headphones and listening. He seemed intrigued by the music and had moments of intense focus. However, he would not leave the headphones on for longer than 2-3 minutes. He never vehemently protested the headphones or became irritable or fussy; rather, he simply removed the headphones and moved on. His response to the music and headphones appeared to be related to the other opportunities available in the environment rather than a dislike of the music.

A second intervention attempted was the introduction of the Wilbarger Touch Pressure Protocol. This protocol is often useful in decreasing sensory defensiveness, improving sensory processing and increasing body awareness. David again seemed intrigued by the application of this technique. He especially seemed to enjoy the joint compression that followed the touch pressure. He did become a little squirmy during use of this technique and it was decided that additional intervention would not be added until a follow-up visit. Additional intervention will include oral-motor strategies.

David, as a 2 year old, seems to present a picture of moderate sensory defensiveness and disregulation. In addition to specific sensory sensitivities and reactivity, David also seems to need intensity of sensory input in order to attain a more regulated state. His difficulties with sleep regu-

> *Instructional Note #5: The process of sound modulation alternately emphasizes the high and low frequencies in the music. This modulation helps the muscles in the middle ear contract and relax, almost as if exercising those muscles. The flexibility of the muscles in the middle ear creates the duality of function of the middle ear: contracting in order to tune in to specific information (e.g. mom's voice over the television) and relaxing in order to monitor the entire environment (e.g. walking in to a new room and noticing all of the sounds before tuning some of them out). In recreating the flexibility of the middle ear, often auditory sensitivities are decreased.*

lation are particularly pronounced. Disregulated sleep is not uncommon for individuals whose overall state regulation is not rhythmical and fluid.

All of David's challenges seem interwoven. Postural organization and integration are difficult to attain due to factors outlined by his physical therapist. He seems to enjoy vestibular and proprioceptive input and these are key in helping to generate a different tonal base. Integration of all systems forms the most solid foundation upon which David can build in order to most easily access the keys to modulation.

Plan

Listening Program
☊ Initiate use of a Therapeutic Listening program with Mozart for Modulation – Modified and Rhythm and Rhyme. Specific instructions were given on a separate form. Follow-up will occur through phone consultation.

Concurrent Treatment Suggestions
✌ The Wilbarger Protocol as demonstrated was recommended 6-8 times per day. "Touch pressure" with deep pressure should always be followed by joint compression.

✌ A Chewy Tube™ was introduced to David. Bits of his preferred foods can be placed in the Chewy Tube for David to chew upon. The placement of the Chewy Tube within David's mouth should gradually be moved toward the back teeth. Only move as far back as possible without eliciting a gag response. Look for a rhythmic chewing response and the ability to chew consecutively. Ideally, a rate of approximately 15 chews/minute would be generated. Chewing can be facilitated by gentle downward pressure on the Chewy Tube (press & release – don't sustain pressure) in the desired rhythm.

✌ A follow-up appointment was scheduled. At this time, David's home program will be updated and more activity suggestions for movement and sensory experiences will be explored.

Name: Jennifer
Age: 4 years

Initial listening program for a
preschooler with pervasive
sensorimotor problems
(see also p. 4-59).

Referral Information

Concerns prompting Jennifer's referral for an occupational therapy consultation included her challenges with sequencing, word retrieval and articulation. Additionally, mild sensory-based issues have been noted as well. For example, Jennifer was 3 years old before she would tolerate a swing. At 4 years old, she still has numerous clothing preferences.

Jennifer was the product of an uncomplicated pregnancy. Early motor milestones were all accomplished within expected intervals. Language milestones have always been slightly delayed. At the age of 18 months, Jennifer had only 8-10 words, by 24 months, this had expanded to only 50-60 words. Jennifer has been a physically healthy child. She has no known allergies and takes no medications.

Jennifer has a history of variable reactivity to sensation. She is very sensitive to how clothes feel on her skin and does not like anything tight around her stomach. She prefers to wear her pants lower than her waist. Seams in her socks also bother her. Shoes or boots that feel too tight are also problematic for Jennifer. She has a history of sensitivity to movement. She now tolerates swinging as long as she can remain in verbal control of the speed, height and direction. She still does not tolerate spinning movement. Jennifer seems to have normal tolerance of sound. As a younger child, she did not seem especially fond of some music. Now, Jennifer seems to miss some sounds or words, fails to attend to what is being said to her, has difficulty copying rhythmic sounds or repeating songs or rhymes and has difficulty following multi-step directions.

Jennifer currently attends preschool. She receives speech therapy services through the public schools in the form of individual therapy and group therapy, each once a week.

Jennifer's parents perceive her strength to be leadership. They see her as being happy, energetic and strong-willed. They are most concerned about her ability to process information, her articulation and her ability to memorize or retain rote sequential skills such as the alphabet, numbers and songs. They're seeking the appropriateness of auditory-based intervention that might help with Jennifer's ability to process information.

Prior to clinical observations in a relatively unstructured environment, several standardized assessments were attempted. Jennifer's attention and ability to follow complex directions impeded her ability to complete a visual perceptual test. A test of auditory discrimination was also initiated but abandoned due to equipment difficulties.

Jennifer obtained a slightly below average score on the VMI. She was able to duplicate horizontal and vertical lines and a circle. She attempted to duplicate a cross and a diagonal line, but some difficulties with spatial organization were apparent. For example, instead of "+," Jennifer drew "F;" she clearly perceived a vertical line with two horizontal lines extending from it, but she could not organize the parts.

Jennifer was also asked to draw a picture of a person. She drew a series of loosely organized circular strokes and lines without any details. She indicated that the top circle was the head, the middle circular marks were the body, two circles below the body were the feet and two lines drawn next to the body were legs (page 4-59).

Jennifer demonstrated a consistent right-handedness. She held the pencil in an immature grasp, with all fingers extended and holding the pencil. This obviously limits distal manipulation of the pencil.

Upon completion of the VMI, a decision was made to introduce EASe Disc 1 as a Therapeutic Listening program for Jennifer. The EASe Disc is modulated music that accentuates the contrast between foreground and background. This should assist Jennifer in distinguishing between relevant and irrelevant auditory information as well as becoming more discriminative or selective regarding the salient details carried in sound (i.e. the differences between an array of consonant sounds). A principle from Tomatis is that the voice can only reproduce what the ear can perceive. The perception and integration of auditory information is listening. While Jennifer's auditory acuity (hearing) has been assessed within normal limits, her ability to listen or accurately perceive sounds within the speech frequencies does not appear to be completely functional.

Jennifer listened to this CD for 30 minutes. Her response was quite notable. Prior to the introduction of headphones, Jennifer had been very chatty, very animated and very physically active. Immediately when she heard the music, she became very still, quiet and focused. It was apparent that she was actively listening. After 15-20 minutes, Jennifer again became more animated, talkative and active. The period of intense internal focus and listening demonstrated by Jennifer is not unusual when modulated music is introduced; this type of response often means the child will be a very good responder to a Therapeutic Listening program.

The middle ear mechanism has a dual function: monitoring the environment (relaxation of the stapedius) and selecting the most salient auditory information (contraction of the stapedius). The stapedius does not seem to functioning with its requisite degree of flexibility to attenuate and focus sound for Jennifer. She seems to have little ability to select out the most rel-

evant or significant information present. Without being able to order and organize information in terms of importance, it will naturally be challenging for Jennifer to learn information largely based on auditory perception (i.e. alphabetic and numeric sequences, the sequences of words in a song).

Jennifer was noted to seek intensity in the types of activities she sought. She was quite comfortable climbing, jumping and crashing. She demonstrated admirable postural control using a trapeze on a zipline. She was able to sustain a flexed upper and lower body position for 20-30 seconds repeatedly while using the trapeze.

Jennifer also immensely enjoyed the lycra hammock swing. She was very comfortable with intense swinging and bouncing in a variety of planes of movement while in the lycra. She did object to having the lycra closed around her, though. Her previously reported caution and dislike of swinging may have had to do with the combination of visual and vestibular input. She seems a bit reliant on visual information to help integrate auditory and vestibular information, thus her dislike of having the lycra closed. However, when the visual information becomes confusing, as it would in a fast moving car or a spinning swing, the vestibular input seems to become disorganizing for Jennifer. This also seems to be especially true when Jennifer cannot add proprioceptive input (resistive input to the muscles and joints inherently provided through activities such as climbing, jumping, pushing, pulling and lifting) to the activity. For example, the lycra swing, regardless of how intense the movement, was acceptable to Jennifer because of the constant feedback provided to her muscles and joints through impact with the lycra. A playground swing or merry-go-round produce little of this same type of input and can become disorganizing for her. She may lose awareness of where her body is in space and feel disoriented and motion sick.

After an intense but highly organized period of movement and exploration, a SAMONAS CD was introduced. The music of Carulli (CQ) was selected because of its intense rhythmicity, which impacts temporal organization. Differences in articulation as well as timing of speech and movement are often observable following use of Carulli. Many of Jennifer's challenges seem related to poor timing and sequencing.

A final intervention technique utilized with Jennifer was the Wilbarger Touch Pressure Protocol. This protocol was initiated with Jennifer due to her history of sensitivity and particularity around clothing. However, her lack of ability to integrate vestibular information in the absence of visual and/or proprioceptive input also made her a good candidate for this technique. The Wilbarger Touch Pressure Protocol increases information to the tactile and proprioceptive systems, thereby enhancing body awareness and connection of the body to the environment.

Jennifer is very reliant on her vision for information. However, vision should be laid upon a foundation created and fortified by the vestibular and auditory systems. The interaction of these three systems is what creates perception. Perception is what gives one an understanding of time and space. If Jennifer cannot filter or distinguish between relevant and irrelevant information with regard to her processing of sensation, the temporal and spatial qualities of many sensory experiences will be lost. In turn, these may lead to challenges with modulation, sequencing, planning and overall organization. When the impact of these challenges is mediated, Jennifer appears to have the tools necessary for competence.

Plan

Listening Program

♪ A Therapeutic Listening program of EASe Disc 1 2x/day for 30 minutes was implemented for Jennifer. This disc was chosen for its sharp contrasts between auditory foreground and background, thereby enhancing its modulatory capacity.

♪ After 3 weeks, CQ 103 (Carulli) will be added to Jennifer's Therapeutic Listening program. This CD should be listened to for 8 minutes 1x/day. She should continue to listen to EASe Disc 1 1x/day for 30 minutes.

♪ Jennifer's listening program will be followed via phone consultation with her parents. A followup appointment will be scheduled as needed.

Concurrent Treatment Suggestions

✍ The Wilbarger Protocol was recommended to be continued 6-8x per day.

✍ An important self-regulator that may be important for Jennifer's general behavioral organization as well as impacting speech and articulation is that of respiration. The idea with any respiratory activity would be to extend the exhalation. Use of blow toys, a bubble tub, or different horns and whistles may hold benefit for Jennifer.

✍ The use of rhythm may also hold great significance for Jennifer in solidifying her processing capacities. When rhythm was used (through movement and voice) in the clinic, Jennifer was able to tell the story of "The Little Mermaid" in a logical sequence while creating a tune of her own in order to tell the story. Rhythm could be used in the form of reciting novel words to familiar nursery rhymes or tunes to give Jennifer instructions, help her with transitions, provide her with information about her day, etc.

For example, singing to the tune of "Are You Sleeping, Brother John?":
> Put your socks on, Put your socks on
> Then your shoes, Then your shoes
> Go and get your backpack
> Go and get your backpack
> Off to school, Off to school

Name: Charlie
Age: 4.6 years

Follow-up of an initial listening program. Severe sensory modulation difficulties warranted a longer period of modulated music followed by a refined SAMONAS program.

Referral Information

Charlie was referred for a Therapeutic Listening assessment due to ongoing concerns regarding his difficulties with modulation and regulation, difficulties with motor planning and difficulties with play and social interaction. In particular, concerns were raised about Charlie's tendency to respond physically (i.e. hitting) when he feels frustrated or overwhelmed or is at a loss for how to otherwise express himself.

Initial Program

Charlie had previously been on a Therapeutic Listening program including modulated music and a SAMONAS Carulli recording. This listening program was initiated by Charlie's occupational and speech therapists. Improved modulation was noted while Charlie was on a Therapeutic Listening program; however, at the time of this assessment, Charlie had not been on a listening program for approximately 4-6 weeks.

Charlie was the product of an uncomplicated pregnancy. At 24 weeks gestation, an ultrasound indicated possible problems in one of the ventricles of the brain; follow-up ultrasound did not substantiate this problem. During birth, some decelerations in the fetal heart rate were recorded but not for a prolonged period. Charlie was born with the umbilical cord around his neck but not so tight as to have caused problems.

Charlie accomplished early motor milestones on the late side of typical. He crawled at 10-12 months and walked independently at 17 months. Language was always more significantly delayed. Charlie had minimal verbal expression by the age of 2. Interestingly, between the ages of 18-24 months, Charlie demonstrated sophisticated fine motor development, eating neatly with utensils and being able to put together beginner puzzles with ease.

According to report, Charlie has fluctuating responses to sensory input, including touch, vision and sound. Tactilely, Charlie was noted to seem sensitive to the tags in shirts. He likes touch when it is "mutually agreed upon" and likes to be cuddled when falling asleep. He shows typical enjoyment of movement experiences but likes to be in control of his own body. Charlie does respond with caution to some movement experiences through space, on unstable surfaces, or involving heights. The sounds of certain toys bother him. At times, he seems to become overstimulated by sound and is sometimes distracted by noises (i.e. telephone) when playing. Sensitivity to light was reported along with difficulty following or tracking with his eyes, avoiding eye contact, having difficulty sustaining visual attention.

Currently, Charlie attends a regular multiage preschool classroom. There, Charlie receives speech services, occupational therapy services and special education services. Primary concerns at school center around Charlie's difficulties with play and socialization. He generally requires adult supervision during play situations; if left unattended, he may become aggressive, hitting, kicking or throwing toys.

Charlie's parents perceive him to be a resilient child with a good sense of humor. He has strong connections to his family and to other familiar people in his life. He is described as usually cheerful, playful and good natured. Charlie's parents are concerned about Charlie's level of anxiety and his difficulties attaining appropriate play and social skills. They worry that he may always have developmental difficulties with his verbal and cognitive skills. They've come to Therapeutic Resources hoping to address the problems of aggression that have escalated recently. They also hope to address difficulties with attention and concentration in order to get Charlie kindergarten ready. Additionally, they hope to gain more tools to address Charlie's modulation.

Assessment/Observations

Though Charlie entered the clinic environment readily, he also demonstrated a fair degree of anxiety. He had anticipated his familiar occupational therapist being present during the session and she had not yet arrived. The novel environment, the unfamiliar adults and the deviance from the expected plan combined to create less than optimal circumstances for Charlie. With all of these factors considered, Charlie adapted as best he could. He had some difficulty sustaining engagement. Though it seemed that he wished to explore the new environment, it also seemed that this choice was too perilous for him given all of the unknowns within the unfamiliar surroundings. Charlie positioned himself so that he could continue to watch for his therapist's arrival. He was more successful participating in activities brought to him at his self-selected lookout place than in attempts to engage him to more broadly explore the space. Once his therapist arrived, Charlie settled more and began to move more freely about the clinic.

When exploring and moving, Charlie sustained the involvement of the adults in the environment. He used a variety of strategies in order to do this. He invited adults directly into his activities; he initiated requests for help when he was challenged by an activity; he summoned attention and interaction by physically connecting with an adult (using both appropriate and aggressive touch).

Charlie was very intrigued by the presence of a peer in the environment. He seemed uncertain of how to initiate interaction with this peer (who was non-verbal and seemed largely unaware of Charlie's presence), though it was clear that he was motivated to do so. He followed this peer around the room, attempting to be in the same space and doing the same activity as the peer. However, due to Charlie's own difficulties with motor planning and language, he was challenged

to connect. Playing in a parallel fashion did not appear to be satisfying; he desired more connection and interaction, yet lacked the tools to be successful with this mission. Because he cannot get to the language of initiation and invitation, he steps in physically. For example, the peer was on a swing. Charlie watched the peer for several seconds then approached. As soon as he came in close physical proximity to the peer, he hit. The intent seemed to be "Hi. Can I play too?" However, even a more responsive peer would likely not interpret the hitting as invitation. Once Charlie has initiated in this way, he seems to feel the wrong of his behavioral choice (which was his most adaptive/available choice in the moment), become frustrated by his lack of success in meeting his goal and his behavior escalates. Again, because he lacks adaptability in his modulation and in his organization and accessibility to language, his behavioral response seems out of proportion to the circumstances, creating a whole energy around others' responses to him and perpetuates a cycle that is familiar to Charlie yet doesn't advance him towards his initial goal of successful interaction with a peer. His desires for interaction and connection appear to be intrinsic and at this moment, he appears ill-equipped to master his intentions. How very reasonable then, to become frustrated, overwhelmed and reactive.

As previously stated, Charlie's difficulties with motor planning appear to contribute to many problematic situations for him. He has the ability to conceive of an idea (i.e. "I want to play with this child," "I want to climb this ladder.") but has decreased ability to develop a plan for achieving the idea. Sometimes this manifests itself as decreased persistence. For example, Charlie attempted to climb an inclined ladder in the clinic many times but was only able to negotiate the first 3 rungs until physically assisted. After climbing 3 rungs, Charlie was near the top of the ladder and needed to move his hands off the ladder and on to the surface of the loft. Charlie did not seem able to actuate a plan for moving from the ladder on to the loft until he was physically assisted. He seemed motivated to climb on the loft and repeatedly attempted to climb the ladder. Neither visual nor verbal assistance were enough for Charlie to be able to follow through on this plan. He seemed to need the feedback from successful repeated motor attempts in order for the plan to hold as well as for emergent generalization of the motor plan into other arenas/activities. So, if Charlie can conceive of, but not develop or execute an idea, then his intentions would be frequently out of sync with the reality created by his actions. His actions and behaviors would often be mismatched to the situation and he may perceive lack of success in many environments. The motoric difficulties could reveal themselves in communication, social initiation and sustained social interaction.

An additional factor for Charlie that seems to contribute to challenges with modulation and behavioral escalation is that his respiratory patterns and suck/swallow/breathe synchrony are poorly organized. Respiration tends to be short, shallow and often arrhythmical, with periods of breath-holding. Short, shallow breathing patterns obligate the nervous system to a high alert state. In this heightened state, it becomes more challenging to grade responses to stimuli in the environment. Behavioral choices tend to be in the form of flight, fright or fight. Poor organization of general oral motor patterns and synergies was also noted. Charlie had difficulty sustaining lip seal on a piece of theratubing and frequently blew the tubing out of his mouth. He also had difficulty differentiating between blowing and sucking - more evidence of his challenges with motor planning. The mouth is a primary organizer of behavior. For Charlie, challenges in this primary level of organization/regulation contribute to larger challenges organizing posture and movement in ways which sustain regulation.

For example, the flight/fright/fight response helps bias Charlie's posture toward use of extension without balanced flexion. The lack of balanced use of flexion with increased movement patterns in extension reinforces movement away and further perpetuates the cycle of flight/fright/fight making it difficult for Charlie to posturally organize and activate in ways that are helpful to him. The heightened state of his nervous system creates a pattern of defensive responses to external touch input that otherwise might prove beneficial for organizing his posture and movement for regulation.

During the assessment, the one time that Charlie tolerated physical touch and handling to assist with postural organization was when touch was introduced in a very playful and novel way. He responded to the unexpected and the humorous. This window of opportunity lasted approximately 10 minutes before the novelty and unpredictability themselves became factors in creating a situation of overwhelm for Charlie. Clearly, this window of opportunity needs to be broadened for Charlie; this is the therapeutic dance.

Finally, Charlie's parents had questions and concerns about strategies to use with Charlie when his behavior escalates and becomes physical. Because the contributing factors are so multi-faceted and because the causative events are myriad and non-identical, developing strategies for helping Charlie and creating change in his behavior has been challenging. While generation of specific ideas is difficult, several principles seem key. First, strategies need to be consistent across environments. This would also mean that expectations should be consistent across environments. It would also seem important that any consequences for behavior should be relatively immediate to the occurrence of the behavior. Though Charlie may be well-versed in the rules, because of the aforementioned challenges, it is doubtful that he can summon them when in the midst of a challenging situation. Additionally, because of Charlie's challenges accessing and organizing language, it may be helpful to reduce the amount of verbiage surrounding explanations, conflict resolution, negotiation, etc. Increasing the non-verbal communication during these times may help with Charlie's ability to process and synthesize the information. One strategy discussed was that of using an 'instant replay.' This strategy essentially allows Charlie to have a do-over of a situation that wasn't successful. An adult can facilitate the 'instant replay' as necessary. In these instances, a sense of humor coupled with as little sense of judgment as possible should be imparted. For example, if Charlie were to push another child, an adult could simply state "Instant Replay!" or "Do-Over!" Then the adult would help Charlie and the other involved child re-enact the sequence of events immediately prior to the pushing incident. Both children will have the opportunity to make different choices to create a different conclusion for the situation.

What appeared to be true for Charlie is that a counter-productive cycle gets set in motion once he perceives a task or situation to be challenging. His escalation seems somewhat disproportionate to the events and then his behavior rather than the source of challenge becomes the focus of attention. His ability to modulate this emotional escalation, especially to determine any strategies for applying the 'brakes' other than shutting down or demonstrating aggressive behaviors, appears quite limited. The challenge is perceived and Charlie immediately rockets into high stress behaviors. This is not to suggest that Charlie is dramatizing or that his challenges with processing sensory information aren't real.

Plan

Listening Program

🎧 A program using modulated music (EASe Disc 1, EASe Disc 2, Rhythm and Rhyme, Mozart for Modulation – Modified) was suggested for Charlie over the next 6-8 weeks. Charlie had good success with this music before and the recent intensification of disregulation suggests that he would benefit from use of the modulated music again. Charlie should listen to these CDs in a random manner, 2x per day, 25-30 minutes each session, at least 3 hours between sessions. While listening, Charlie should be engaged in low stress, low verbal activities.

The use of Sounds of Nature (ST 110), a SAMONAS CD was introduced. Charlie's listening time is 1x/day for 5 minutes followed by one of his sessions of modulated music. This CD was selected to help broaden Charlie's awareness of space and perhaps become more adept at moving through it with gradation and planning.

Finally, it was suggested that during his speech and OT sessions (which occur a total of 4x/week), Charlie listen to Classic (CQ 101) for approximately 10 minutes while also engaging in oral motor activities. Classic was suggested to address issues surrounding disorganization of respiration and suck/swallow/breathe.

Concurrent Treatment Suggestions

✎ If Charlie is to have success with self-regulation, his school schedule must be reflective of his needs. While Charlie appears to have good days and bad days at school, it is this very inconsistency that bears addressing. Regardless of how his day might be labeled in terms of his ability to self-regulate and remain organized and focused within the classroom, it will be important to have routine breaks throughout the day.

✎ Respiratory activities can be used to connect eyes to hands to facilitate eye-hand coordination. Blow toys with moving parts help the eyes work together. Additionally, using theratubing to vary the length that the blow toy is from the eyes helps to create opportunities for the eyes to work together in different ranges and planes of motion. Different diameters and shapes of mouth pieces should be used with Charlie as well to help him practice generating adequate lip seal. (See pg. 3-73.)

✎ Postural organization should be a key modulator for Charlie. The challenge with Charlie is finding ways to introduce movement activities using the principles (weight bearing with alignment, rotation, diaphragmatic breathing, balanced flexion with extension) without setting up a defensive or disregulated response. Much as a floortime model suggests 6-8X20-30 minutes interludes of floortime per day, Charlie should have 6-8X5-10 minutes of posturally organizing activity per day. Postural activities can be followed by respiratory activities to lengthen the periods of modulation/regulation gained.

✎ Specific oral motor activities were shared with Charlie's OT during the assessment. These activities should be part of Charlie's ongoing treatment program/therapy sessions.

Referral Information

Concerns prompting Chloe's referral for an occupational therapy intensive included her challenges with motor skills, attention span, speech apraxia and general rate of learning and acquisition of new skills. Chloe receives a multitude of therapies in her home community including speech therapy, occupational therapy, physical therapy and tutoring for reading.

Initial Program

Prior to her initial visit at Therapeutic Resources, Chloe had been on a Therapeutic Listening program for almost 4 months. Chloe had listened to EASe Disc 2 for 2 weeks at which time her original therapist discontinued use of modulated music. For the past 4 months, she has listened to Carulli in a CQ format for 2 half hours per day. This is an unusually long listening time, even on a CQ SAMONAS. However, for Chloe, the gains were tremendous. She began to read phonetically, her drawings and writing showed significantly more refinement, she ceased to require as much intense movement to promote concentration and attention and she was able to filter out some commotion in the environment. Chloe's parents are interested in pursuing the next step for her.

Chloe was the product of a normal pregnancy. Delivery was complicated by a prolonged labor lasting 41 hours. After delivery, she needed a little oxygen intermittently. She was described as being an irritable and sensitive infant. Motor milestones were all accomplished on the late side of typical. Chloe sat alone at 8 months, crawled at 11 months, turned over at 11 months and walked at 16 months. Chloe hated being on her stomach when she was a baby and would scream until her position was changed. Language was always significantly delayed.

Chloe has a history of significant sensitivity or reactivity to sensation, though the extremeness of her sensitivity has resolved substantially as she has grown older and received ongoing interventions. Chloe used to be so sensitive to sounds that she would have to sit down in the presence of loud noises; the noises literally knocked her off of her feet. Additionally, in a noisy or busy environment, Chloe has difficulty focusing. Though much improved, this is still a challenge for her. She reportedly used to be quite sensitive to many touch sensations though this is no longer an issue. Chloe reportedly uses movement to organize, although she has mild fear of movement through space. Additionally, she is quite sensitive to light.

Chloe's parents perceive her strengths to be her extremely happy disposition, her positive attitude, her positive self-esteem and her willingness to work hard and keep trying. They are concerned about her developmental lags, though she has made wonderful progress, particularly in the last year. They want to protect Chloe's self-esteem while helping her realize her fullest potential. They are very encouraged by the results they have had from Chloe's Therapeutic Listening program and have come to Therapeutic Resources seeking the 1what's next with regards to a listening program as well as any other interventions or strategies that might be useful for Chloe.

Observation/Assessment

During the initial hour of Chloe's intensive, a variety of standardized assessments were administered with the following results:

Chloe achieved consistent performance on all of the subtests of the VMI. Her performance level was in the slightly below average range (a standard score of 85 would have been low average). While at this time her performance is below age level expectation, the evenness of her performance is encouraging as it suggests parallel development and integration of her sensory systems (i.e. as information from her senses becomes organized and integrated, Chloe is able to demonstrate functional skill with that information).

Chloe demonstrated a right hand preference. She held the pencil in a digital pronated grasp with little isolated finger movement observed during writing. She continues to direct the motion of the pencil across the paper from her shoulder. She also holds her jaw and tongue in retraction when writing in order to recruit additional stability.

Sequencing and spatial organization appear to be areas of challenge for her. She omitted the initial "e" in her name when writing it but did visually inspect her work and self-correct her error. Additionally, it was observed that Chloe often initiates writing and drawing from bottom-to-top and from right-to-left.

From Chloe's history, auditory sensitivity and discrimination were reported to be areas of significant challenge for her. This certainly proved true on the Test of Auditory Discrimination. On both the Quiet and Noise (noisy background such as in a school cafeteria) Subtests, Chloe struggled. While Chloe appeared to be actively exerting her best effort on the Quiet Subtest, she became noticeably stressed during the Noise Subtest. Her skin flushed, her eyes began to lose focus and she appeared to be guessing.

Chloe's middle ear mechanism does not appear to be functioning with the expected level of flexibility (refer to Instructional Note #2, pg. 4-4). It may be difficult for her to create an appropriate balance between auditory foreground and background, thus focusing on specific auditory information (i.e. the teacher's voice) with accuracy may be challenging. Chloe may become overstimulated in 'busy' auditory environments

and tune out. For Chloe, it appears that her ears are 'open' at all times and sound is perceived as if directly on top of her. Therefore, in busier or noisier environments, the density of information may overwhelm her. Additionally, if the auditory information is all perceived as 'foreground,' Chloe is not discriminating the spatial information carried in sound. This would be reflected in her motor skills such as competence on dynamic surfaces or even in the spatial qualities of her handwriting.

Subtle, qualitative differences were noted in Chloe's postural organization and movement. In stationary positions or in movement, Chloe seemed to rely on a wide base of support. She kept her extremities positioned outward from her body in order to recruit additional stability. She did not demonstrate fluid bilateral integration/coordination or midline orientation/organization. These patterns are necessary before more refined movement patterns, such as movement across midline and in rotation (around the body center), can be consistently demonstrated and accessed. As is true for many children with similar subtle postural issues, Chloe was more confident using her lower extremities than her upper extremities and tended to avoid truly activating her upper extremities by finding another way to move. For example, when climbing up through a trap door in a loft, Chloe would place her arms on the upper level and push with her legs from the lower level until she had maneuvered most of her body through the hole. She would not push onto or bear weight on her upper extremities unless facilitated. Her movement was biased toward extension and she lacked nice dynamic balance between flexion and extension.

From a sensory integrative perspective, it would seem that Chloe's vestibular system is not 'turning on' efficiently. Chloe uses the external environment to provide herself with knowledge of where she is in space. She relies on her mother for external referencing. She also uses her visual system to provide spatial awareness and understanding as best she can without sufficient integration and input from the vestibular and auditory systems. Her uncertain relationship to gravity was still apparent. While she could demonstrate fearless behavior, she also demonstrated a great deal of caution at times. For instance, she quickly darted away from any rough and tumble play. Any time she was on the ground, she sought to keep her head in an upright position, often placing her body in awkward positions in order to maintain that upright position. If her vestibular system is not providing feedback efficiently, then it will be important for Chloe to maintain a head position that gives her an unvaried orientation to the horizon. Change her head position, her orientation to the horizon changes and she no longer is certain where she is in space.

Instructional Note #6: *The vestibular system is important in defining one's relationship to gravity and also providing the reference point of where one is in space. The vestibular system has diffuse connections to other lower centers in the brain including the reticular formation (regulates arousal, attention, alertness) and the limbic system (emotional tone). The vestibular system, through its connections with the cerebellum, also plays a role in mediating postural tone and coordinating movement. Because of its bilateral representation, the vestibular system is especially important in helping coordinate the two sides of the body.*

Finally, while Chloe was at Therapeutic Resources, an intensive oral motor program using exercises developed by Debra Beckman, MS, CCC-SLP, was initiated. The exercises facilitated more mobility and less tension in all of the perioral tissues, including cheeks, lips and nasal area. Chloe responded very favorably to these exercises, with subsequent differences in her facial appearance noted. Continuance of these exercises should help with articulation.

Interpretation

Chloe is very reliant on her external senses, especially her visual sense; however, her visual system cannot stand alone (see Instructional Note #4, pg. 4-9). It should be laid upon a foundation created and fortified by the vestibular and auditory systems. The interaction of these systems is what creates perception. Perception is what gives one an understanding of time and space. If Chloe is truly in the 'sensory soup' with regard to her processing of sensation, the temporal and spatial qualities of many sensory experiences will be lost.

Chloe does not seem to be organized in space and time because she does not perceive them in the dimensionality or wholeness that would be typical. Without an understanding of the three-dimensionality of space, Chloe cannot efficiently move through it nor will she seek to move her body in ways that challenge gravity and refine her movement and postural organization. It is not surprising, then, that she holds her head in a constant orientation in order to maintain constancy in her spatial understanding of the environment. It is also not surprising that she demonstrates caution in attempting novel movement experiences or when some of her control regarding her movement experiences is threatened.

Additionally, Chloe does not seem to have a clear understanding of time. She can demonstrate slight delays in her responses to input, especially auditory input. She often verbally repeats information or questions "what?" as strategies to buy time in order to process information more successfully.

Plan

Listening Program
♁ A Therapeutic Listening program of ST 110 and ST 101 was implemented with Chloe. ST 110 was selected for the spatial qualities present in the context of the nature. ST 101 was chosen for its rhythmical simplicity in providing a framework for higher levels of attention and organization, especially around primary rhythms such as coordination or synchronization of suck/swallow/breathe.

♁ Additionally, Chloe's Therapeutic Listening program will include use of the Baroque for Modulation – Modified 2x day for 30 minutes each session to continue to promote modulation of sensory information. After a two week period Mozart Strings will be added to continue to promote modulation and proper middle ear function.

Concurrent Treatment Suggestions

🖐 The use of a Therapeutic Listening program often 'opens the window' for emergent functional skill. In Chloe's case, postural control must be activated before significant changes in movement and skill are noted. Otherwise, Chloe will continue to swim upstream and likely become increasingly frustrated by her efforts.

🖐 Please refer to pg. 3-42 for ideas regarding postural organization.

🖐 Respiratory activities will be important as part of Chloe's program. Positioning during respiratory activities is also important. Ideally, Chloe should be in a position that is providing pressure to and thus activating her diaphragm. Swinging in prone is one option (provided that the surface of the swing is around her trunk and not under her arms). Sitting back on her heels with her trunk flexed forward (perhaps blowing through tubing into a bubble tub) is another way to maintain pressure to the diaphragm.

🖐 Respiratory activities can also be used to obtain more focused, central vision. Blow toys with moving parts help the eyes work together. Using theratubing to vary the length that the blow toy is from the eyes helps to create opportunities for the eyes to work together in different ranges and planes of motion. These activities can be teamed with Chloe's listening session.

🖐 A variety of specific structured oral-motor activities based upon Debra Beckman's work were implemented while Chloe was at the clinic. These exercises were demonstrated to her parents and should be continued at home 1-2x daily. Specific exercises included upper and lower cheek stretches, gum massage, upper and lower lip stretches, upper and lower lip curls and stretching of the entire nasal area. "Stretching" in this context refers to myofascial release or waiting for the tissues to respond and relax rather than a forceful stretch against resistance.

Name: Jane R.
Age: 5.11 years

Modification of a listening program after one year with an initial listening protocol.

Referral Information

Difficulties with peer relationships as well as challenges with modulation prompted Jane's referral for an occupational therapy consultation. Jane attends a typical preschool classroom and her teachers feel that her development is not far from her age-mates but that she needs help redirecting her attention. She is academically prepared for kindergarten in the 2001-2002 school year, but she is challenged socially; she cannot hold a spontaneous conversation with peers and her play schemes can be repetitive and limited.

Jane is involved in intensive intervention in her home community. She receives ongoing occupational therapy and speech therapy services. Her family works with a psychologist. She receives in-home floortime therapy.

Initial Program

At the time of this consultation at Therapeutic Resources, Jane had been on a Therapeutic Listening program for approximately one year. During that time, she had listened to a variety of modulated music (EASe Disc 1, EASe Disc 2, EASe Disc 4 and Mozart for Modulation – Modified). She had also listened to Carulli in a CQ format and Sounds of Nature. Her maximum listening time to either SAMONAS CD was 20 minutes. Throughout the duration of her listening program, she maintained at least 30 minutes per day of modulated music.

Initial changes observed with modulated music (prior to the introduction of SAMONAS) included:
- increased availability and engagement.
- less constant oral craving and mouthing.
- greater connectedness to the environment.
- consistency with toilet training.

After 4 months on modulated music alone, Carulli was introduced (as suggested in the protocol– 5 minutes per day, adding 1 minute every 4th day) and additional changes were noted:

- decreased toe walking.
- increased jaw stability.
- improvements in motor planning– e.g. negotiating a variety of surfaces and equipment in the environment.
- improvements in rhythmicity and bilaterality of movement.

After 3 months on Carulli, Sounds of Nature was introduced and Carulli was no longer used in Jane's program. With the addition of Sounds of Nature, Jane showed the following gains:

- improved spatial awareness.
- better 1:1 relating to people and objects within the environment.
- more fluid movement through space.
- better understanding of middle and distant visual space.
- improved function in a classroom situation with respect to peer orientation and ability to follow classroom routine.

Jane's parents perceive her strengths to be her happy nature, her sense of humor and her creativity when playing with her toy characters. They've come to explore any additional avenues for intervention with Jane. In preparation for her kindergarten year, Jane's parents want to pinpoint areas of greatest concern and address those whole-heartedly in the coming months.

Jane entered the clinic enthusiastically. She was comforted by the presence of her familiar occupational and speech therapists. She was able to explore fairly independently. Her initial responses depicted a mild state of disorganization, with rote, silly responses to questions and conversation and more scripted play that was hard to interrupt or re-route.

Because a primary concern regarding Jane's ability to remain contextually in a conversation, Therapeutic Listening CDs selected were geared toward this challenge. The timing and interplay of responding seem difficult for Jane, so the music of Mozart (CQ 108) was selected because of its conversational dynamics (call and response; echoing of a varied theme). Jane easily accepted the music.

Only mild disregulation was seen in the session, implying that Jane is able to maintain basic regulation quite effectively most of the time and that her needs are more in higher-level self-regulation. Toward this end, a variety of strategies were attempted, including use of another SAMONAS CD (CQ 104 – Live in Catalunya/ Chamber Music).

Jane responded very positively to a number of different strategies. She seemed to be initiating use of her mouth as one means of self-regulation. Continued oral stimulation as well as maximizing use of oral strategies across environments would be useful for Jane. In the clinic, use of a kazoo, sour tastes, cold temperatures, and resistive suck were all organizing for her.

Additionally, Jane's eyes are not always connected to her movement through an environment. She seems to either visually monitor or visually overfocus. When she moves through space, she sights then moves, sights then moves. Reducing her visual space (i.e. the lycra swing) helped this significantly. However, creating opportunities for postural organization with orientation toward midline helped organize her vision as well. Again, use of the kazoo, use of resistive sucking, as well as heavy work patterns with alignment of joints and resistance to movement served her well.

Jane is progressing beautifully. She has a number of strategies that seem successful for her

in maintaining a more regulated state much of the time. Challenges remain in Jane's ability to self-regulate across environments in a way which allows her to maintain engagement with others in a reciprocal, mutually-driven manner.

For Jane, self-regulation is certainly a matter of refinement of strategies that she is already attempting to employ. She attempts to use her mouth as a means of self-regulation. She attempts to use movement in flexion (rocking on her hands and knees) as a means to self-regulate. She needs assistance making these strategies more precise and more appropriately accessible regardless of the environment. She seems ready to begin the more cognitive process of identifying strategies for self-regulation.

An additional avenue to explore with Jane is that of the vestibular-visual connection to see if greater connection of vision to movement can be accessed. She doesn't always use her eyes in a more graded manner to sustain connection with her environment or with another person.

Plan

Listening Program

◑ Jane has been on a Therapeutic Listening program under the guidance of her occupational and speech therapists. She has made nice gains using CDs for modulation, for timing and for spatial awareness.

◑ Based upon the goals desired and the challenges presented by Jane during the assessment, her Therapeutic Listening program was modified as follows:

◑ Her first listening session of the day should be Mozart & Contemporaries (CQ 108) for 10 minutes followed by Live in Catalunya (CQ 104) for 10 minutes. Mozart & Contemporaries was selected to address conversational flow as well as higher level processing issues. Live in Catalunya was selected to address refinement of regulation.

◑ Her second listening session of the day should be an EASe disc or Mozart-Modified for 30 minutes. Because Jane has been on these CDs for an extended period of time, it will be important to keep variety in the use of these CDs so that she does not habituate.

◑ Because Jane has gained much through the use of other SAMONAS CDs, these will likely be woven back into her program once her response to this program is known.

Concurrent Treatment Suggestions

✌ The Wilbarger protocol was recommended to be continued 2-3x per day.

✌ Respiratory activities were recommended to begin each treatment with Jane. The specific activities can take an infinite number of forms. The key considerations should be maintaining a flexed position, emphasizing graded exhalation and postural and visual orientation toward midline.

✌ See pages 3-44 to 3-49 for suggestions related to postural activation.

✌ Beginning to teach Jane the concepts of self-regulation will be an important step, particularly as she readies for kindergarten. The concepts, as laid out in the book "How Does Your Engine Run?: The Alert Program for Self-Regulation" (Williams & Shellenberger) can lend themselves nicely to Jane's current therapy regimen. They meld well with both a sensory processing model and a Greenspan approach.

Name: Emily
Age: 4.4 years

Refinement of a listening program for a preschooler following an inital protocol.

Referral Information

Concerns prompting Emily's referral for an occupational therapy consultation included her difficulties with peer relationships and socialization. She is described as a child who has difficulty with modulation; contextually, she understands the extremes or poles and is challenged to understand the in-between. Her challenges with understanding and internalizing more subtle dynamic processes are reflected behaviorally; she tends to be an intense, reactive child.

Initial Program

Prior to her appointment at Therapeutic Resources, Emily had been on a program of modulated music (EASe Disc 1, EASe Disc 2 and Mozart for Modulation – Modified, Rhythm & Rhyme) for approximately 6 months. She has also listened to Carulli CQ and Sounds of Nature which have been blended with modulated CDs. While improvements in Emily's modulation had been observed on the modulated music, she had also developed insistent, rigid patterns about how the CDs were used (i.e. which CD had to be listened to first, which songs she would listen to). Because the changes observed with the modulated music seemed subtler in nature, the question addressed during Emily's initial consultation was regarding the use of any particular music to unstick her tendencies toward rigidity.

Emily is involved in intensive intervention in her home community. She receives ongoing occupational therapy and speech therapy services. Her family works with a psychologist. Additionally, she receives consultation with Stanley Greenspan and Serena Wieder every 6 months. Emily is enrolled in a typical preschool setting and has a designated aide to assist her in the classroom.

Emily's parents perceive her strengths to be her ability to understand things and learn quickly. They state that she is able to derive pleasure from her experiences. They also say that though she can become extremely agitated, she calms down quickly and is able to overcome her fears. They've come for information to fine-tune her current therapeutic regimen.

Emily entered the clinic in what was described to be a typical manner. She was curious and excited about the new environment. However, she demonstrated clear avoidance behaviors as well, verbally expressing her dislike of things while still willingly exploring and interacting. At times, there was a definite mismatch between Emily's verbalizations and her actions.

Emily explored the clinic using familiar toys (brought from home) to assist her. The toys seemed to provide range to her affective expression. They also seemed to provide motivation for her to explore unfamiliar or uncomfortable territory. Once Emily had created a play scenario using her Blues Clues™ toys, the scenario could be modified and manipulated to facilitate greater variety and exploration of movement as well as to create possibilities for more problem solving, more expression and more resolution of intense emotional states.

When Emily's intended scenario was modified, she was initially tolerant and even intrigued. However, as the challenge was increased and the game repeated, Emily became progressively more upset and frustrated. The frustration seemed to be due to an internal perception that she would not be successful in managing the challenge presented. Once the challenge was mastered, Emily quickly recovered. With each repeated thwart to her plans, Emily's emotional upset became greater. At no time during the repetition of the one game (which lasted perhaps

30 minutes) did Emily fail to recover or fail to succeed in completing the task.

As Emily fatigued, her resilience naturally became less. She became more insistent on the rules and more insistent on maintaining control. She was still willing to participate in a novel activity provided she was able to determine all of the other factors surrounding the activity (i.e. who would participate with her, the sequence of the activity).

Much of Emily's disregulation with activity appeared to be related to inefficient sensory processing and its subsequent outcomes for her. In particular, the vestibular-auditory-visual triad appears to be poorly integrated and modulated. For Emily, vestibular inefficiency is seen in postural weakness, especially through the upper extremities. Additional signs are the ease with which she becomes emotionally disregulated and the challenges she faces sustaining a more optimal arousal state in which flexibility of interaction is available to her.

The efficiency of the auditory and visual systems is laid upon the foundation provided by the vestibular system. It is integration of the vestibular-auditory-visual systems that provide one with one's own unique perceptual map. Integration of the three systems gives meaning and dimension to time and space. The ability to read and respond to subtleties of affect and social nuance are dependent upon organization in time and space. More concretely, skills such as throwing and catching a ball are dependent upon organization in time and space. Catching a ball is dependent upon understanding where one's own body is in space, where the ball is in relationship to one's body, the path of the ball as it travels through space and coordinating the timing of one's body with the movement of the ball through space in order to catch.

Clearly, other factors influence Emily's performance as well. She has a highly reactive or sensitive nervous system. The balance between the protective and discriminative functions of her nervous system is skewed toward protection. When this is true, less energy is available for discriminative tasks as more energy is used for monitoring and protection. In the example of catching the ball, Emily's visual energy is often used for surveying and monitoring the environment for possible threat; therefore, she is unable to remain visually focused on the ball.

Instructional Note #7: *The vestibular system is the reference point against which all other sensation is measured. The vestibular system provides a sense of where one's body is in space as well as defining one's relationship to gravity. Among other functions, the vestibular system is important in activating and mediating postural tone and regulating arousal states. Through its ties with the limbic system, it also plays a role in emotional regulation.*

The vestibular influences on postural tone affect Emily's performance as well. Without the vestibular system efficiently mediating postural tone, it is difficult for Emily to get her body in an appropriate state of readiness to master a task. Again, the example of catching a ball: Emily has difficulty sustaining the dynamic cocontraction around her shoulder girdles needed in order to maintain a postural state of readiness to catch a ball.

Finally, integrating these pieces is the challenge of praxis. Praxis is the ability to conceptualize, create a plan for and execute a motor task. In the clinic, Emily was clearly able to ideate. However, developing a plan of action (which involves sequencing, timing, grading and a myriad of other processes) is more challenging for her. Her perception is astute enough for her to see a motor challenge and immediately respond to that challenge with an attitude of success or failure. Her ability to problem solve successfully is a stumbling block for her. She has developed a host of useful strategies in order to compensate for this challenge. Chief among her strategies is remaining in control and determining the rules.

Plan

Listening Program

ᴖ Emily has been on a Therapeutic Listening program under the guidance of her occupational and speech therapists. She has made nice gains using CDs for modulation, for timing (CQ 103) and for spatial awareness (ST 110).

ᴖ What seems true for Emily is that the pieces are all available, but integrating them remains the challenge. Hindering her performance is the emotional coding that accompanies challenges she perceives as "too much." It would be useful to help Emily move through this emotion rather than escaping it by something or someone external resolving the conflict for her.

ᴖ To that end, her Therapeutic Listening program was modified as follows:

ᴖ Her listening time was decreased to one session per day. She will listen to Romantic (CQ 102) for 10 minutes followed by the use of either an EASe disc or Mozart-Modified for 20 minutes. Emily's progress will be followed via phone consultation and modifications made as necessary.

ᴖ Because Emily has gained much through the use of other SAMONAS and modulated CDs, these will likely be woven back into her program once her response to Romantic is known.

Concurrent Treatment Suggestions

✍ The Wilbarger protocol was recommended to be continued 2-3x per day.

✍ Respiratory activities were recommended to begin each treatment with Emily. The specific activities can take an infinite number of forms. The key considerations should be maintaining a flexed position, emphasizing graded exhalation and postural and visual orientation toward midline.

✍ See pages 3-44 to 3-49 for suggestions related to postural activation.

✍ A treatment intensive at Therapeutic Resources in order to challenge Emily's postural development, coordination of vestibular-visual responses and refinement of higher level praxis skills is also recommended.

Name: Bennett
Age: 7.9 years

Refining an extended Therapeutic Listening™ program including integration with other professional services.

Referral Information

Concerns prompting Bennett's referral for an occupational therapy consultation included his challenges with modulation, communication, socialization and ability to read non-verbal cues.

Initial Program

Bennett had been on a Therapeutic Listening program since the fall of 2000. His program consisted primarily of modulated CDs. He also used two SAMONAS CDs in the CQ format (Cadaques Night and Classic). Changes noted in Bennett's skills and behaviors since beginning Therapeutic Listening include increased communication and eye contact and increased flexibility and flow. Refinement of Bennett's listening program was the primary consideration of this occupational therapy consultation.

Bennett is involved in intensive intervention in his home community. He receives ongoing occupational therapy and speech therapy services. His family works with a psychologist. Additionally, Bennett is enrolled in public school and has a 1:1 aide to assist with mainstreaming. Bennett also receives support services of OT and speech therapy to assist him in his school environment.

Bennett has a history of variable reactivity or sensitivity to sensation as well as fluctuation in his ability to effectively integrate and organize sensation for use. He reportedly is slightly less tolerant of touch than typical. He likes movement but will avoid fast rides. Bennett has difficulty filtering relevant from irrelevant auditory stimuli and can be easily distracted by both auditory and visual stimuli. He is reported to have difficulty listening if others are talking, processing multistep directions and attending to what is said to him. Additionally, Bennett is a strong visual learner but is challenged by a moving visual field.

Bennett's parents perceive his strengths to be his outgoing and gregarious nature and his intelligence. They also note that Bennett has the ability to memorize many things. They are concerned about Bennett's difficulties with understanding other people's emotions and feelings. They state that he has difficulty reading non-verbal cues. They would like him to learn more awareness of others. They've come seeking information about how to update Bennett's listening program as well as any interventions or strategies that might be useful for Bennett in increasing his physical, social and emotional regulation.

Assessment/Observations

Prior to clinical observations of Bennett's posture, movement, modulation and organization in a less structured environment, the Test for Auditory Processing Disorders in Children (SCAN-C) was administered.

Bennett scored in the low average range on the Filtered Words subtest and below average on the remainder of the subtests of the SCAN-C. He became increasingly disorganized as the testing progressed. The first indicator that Bennett was losing modulation was decreased clarity in his articulation. He began to swallow the ends of his words and his pronunciation quickly disintegrated into mostly vowel sounds. As he continued to lose modulation, Bennett became increasingly motorically restless, had difficulty sustaining connection to the examiner or to the process and began to subvocalize.

On the *Competing Sentences* subtest, Bennett struggled considerably. On this subtest, a sentence is spoken into each ear, with one sentence being given more volume than the other. The instructions are to repeat the sentence in a specific ear (whichever one has been given more volume). Bennett attempted to say all of the words presented in each ear, with the result being a non-meaningful jumble of words.

For Bennett, the more busy , competing, or intense the auditory environment, the more likely he may become disregulated. Without being able to order and organize information in terms of importance, he responds as if everything is important. Stress and fatigue will likely result from this pattern of response; eventually, Bennett may simply shut down or tune out.

So, it is not surprising that Bennett has difficulty with sports. There are multiple parts to manage, much of the instruction is verbal and is presented as Bennett is in motion and the space keeps shifting and changing as all of the players move. Additionally, dependent on the arena in which the sport is being played, parts of the sound may be faultily transmitted. Indoor sports facilities have poor acoustics that muffle and distort sound. Dependent upon the size of an outdoor playing field, sound may also be lost if the speaker is at a distance from Bennett. He might perceive cars on the road, dogs barking and other peripheral noise as of equal volume and importance as a speaker's voice.

General Observations

Upon completion of the SCAN-C, a decision was made to introduce Baroque-Modified as a Therapeutic Listening program for Bennett. The Baroque-Modified is modulated music; inherent in the structure of baroque compositions is high contrast. For Bennett, the element of high contrast coupled with the accentuation of auditory foreground/background provided by the modulation of the music should help train the ear to be more selective and discriminative.

Bennett listened to this CD for 30 minutes while moving freely about the clinic environment, exploring different spaces and pieces of

> *Instructional Note: #8: The middle ear mechanism has a dual function: monitoring the environment (relaxation of the stapedius) and selecting the most salient auditory information (contraction of the stapedius). The stapedius does not seem to functioning with its requisite degree of flexibility to attenuate and focus sound for Bennett. All information seems to be perceived as foreground with little ability to select out the most relevant or significant information present.*

equipment. It was noted that following use of the Baroque-Modified, Bennett seemed more regulated, more interactive and better able to spontaneously initiate a greater variety of activities in the clinic.

Following a short period of movement in the clinic, the music of Carulli was introduced (in a CQ format) over headphones. Carulli was selected because of its intense rhythmicity, which impacts temporal organization. Differences in articulation as well as timing of speech and movement are often observable following use of Carulli.

While listening, Bennett opted to position himself in a barrel. While in the barrel, a taste picnic was introduced. Intensely sour or spicy flavored candies were used for the taste picnic. By increasing the intensity of oral input, it was hoped that Bennett's range of facial expressiveness would also be increased. While Bennett remained engaged and participatory during the taste picnic, he would not sample anything with which he was unfamiliar. He preferred intensely sour tastes (like Warheads®). Though his face clearly registered the extremeness of the taste (to the point of eyes watering), Bennett did not verbally express that the taste was sour.

Following the 10-minute interlude of Carulli and the taste picnic, Bennett seemed to become a little disregulated. His speech became less contextual and more scripted or rote. His affect was high and a little giddy . His repetition of seemingly nonsensical words was used as an invitation to play in ways that promoted heavy work and respiratory strategies in order to increase Bennett's ability to maintain a modulated state. This period and intensity of play was easily sustained for 20-30 minutes. Initially, Bennett demonstrated approach-avoid behaviors regarding the intensity of the physical contact. However, he did keep repeating and inviting through his words. Because it seemed as though Bennett's language is not always his most useful and specific means of communication, a kazoo was introduced. The kazoo provided an avenue for taking Bennett out of the language that seemed to perpetuate a slightly disorganized cycle of behavior. The kazoo was also selected because of its vibratory resonance, which is very self-regulating. Bennett was immediately intrigued by the kazoo and used it to promote self-regulation even after the game had finished.

Bennett was able to complete the session in a very organized manner. He was able to play independently and quietly for a period of 15-20 minutes while the adults present discussed the events of the day.

Interpretation

The visual and auditory systems form two-thirds of a sensorimotor triad. The vestibular system is the remaining element of this triad which can be likened to the tripod of a camera. The vestibular system responds to gravity and plays a large role in balance, mediation of postural tone and overall state regulation and level of arousal. The vestibular sense is the sense against which all other senses are referenced. However, if any component of the vestibular-visual-auditory triad is weak, inefficient, or impaired, the other components are affected as well. It is the manner in which the triad functions and integrates that defines one's perception. Bennett is very reliant on his external senses for information. However, these should be laid upon a foundation created and fortified by the vestibular system. The interaction of the visual/auditory & vestibular systems is what creates perception. Perception is what gives one an understanding of time and space. If Bennett cannot filter or distinguish between relevant and irrelevant information with regard to his processing of sensation, the temporal and spatial qualities of many sensory experiences will be lost. In turn, these may lead to challenges with modulation, sequencing, planning and overall organization.

Plan

Listening Program

◗ A Therapeutic Listening program of Baroque—Modified 1x/day for 30 minutes was implemented for Bennett. This disc was chosen for its sharp contrasts between auditory foreground and background. Several additional recommendations for a second listening session per day were recommended, based upon the therapy service that Bennett receives that day.

◗ Chamber Music/Live in Catalunya (CQ)—not to exceed 10 minutes listening time; use in speech therapy or OT for sequencing, respiration, self-regulation.

◗ Sounds of Nature—not to exceed 10 minutes listening time; use in OT for enhancing spatial awareness.

◗ Romantic Flute, Harp, & Cello (CQ) — not to exceed 10 minutes listening time; use in speech therapy or with Mom for expression, engagement, broadening affective range.

◗ On days when Bennett does not have an afternoon therapy, he could listen to the Baroque CD for a second 30-minute session.

◗ It was also recommended that Bennett use Carulli as part of a home Therapeutic Listening program. It was recommended that his listening time begin at 5 minutes and that he not remain on Carulli for longer than 2 weeks without consultation regarding its impact occurring. Use of Carulli should not begin until Bennett has listened to the Baroque CD for at least 2 weeks.

Concurrent Treatment Suggestions

✍ The use of a Therapeutic Listening program often opens the window for emergent functional skill. In Bennett's case, postural control must be activated before significant changes in movement and skill are noted. Otherwise, Bennett will continue to swim upstream and likely become increasingly frustrated by his efforts.

✎   See pages 3-44 to 3-49 for ideas regarding postural organization.

✎   An important self-regulator that Bennett has not begun to effectively exploit is that of respiration. The idea with any respiratory activity would be to extend the exhalation. Use of blow toys, a bubble tub, or different horns and whistles may hold benefit for Bennett. He was quite captivated by a kazoo and this was especially helpful as it helped move him away from his scripted language. The bone conduction generated by the kazoo also helps to increase self-regulation.

✎   Finally, since sustaining self-regulation throughout the school day is a great challenge for Bennett, possibilities for enhancing the therapeutic elements of transitions or academic activities were discussed. Several ideas include:

➢   Use of a cloth tunnel for crawling from place to place from a room, or crawling through to gather materials for a next activity.
➢   Use of a bubble tub for blowing for a few minutes between scheduled activities.
➢   Use of a straw with bingo chips for use during assorted academic tasks.

Name: Sara
Age: 6 years

Eileen Hamele, MS, CCC-SLP, Madison, WI

Integrating Therapeutic Listening into speech/language programming - from the Speech/ Language Pathologist's perspective

As a speech and language therapist with nearly 15 years experience, I have yet to use a tool that has been more effective than Therapeutic Listening. Having these powerful tools has completely changed the scope and success of my practice. "Body" is a word I find myself using quite frequently as I explain my goals and music selection to the families with whom I work. Over the years practicing speech, in conjunction with occupational therapy and Sensory Integration, the connection between the body and speech and language has become clearer to me.

I recently had the pleasure of evaluating a beautiful seven-year-old girl whose parents have questioned her speech and language skills since approximately 18 months of age. Sara's mother reports that Sara didn't lose her speech but noted her development slowed at approximately 15-18 months of age. Sara is a first grader who attends a private school, but is not currently receiving any support services through her school. She has received services through a modified Applied Behavioral Analysis program for the past several years. Her parents are concerned about whether Sara will be able to keep up with her classmates as the challenges of school increase. They identify her challenges as not knowing labels for objects and using poor sentence formation. She also has social challenges, including not initiating eye contact or responding to verbal information in a timely manner. Sara may be responding to one question, but her communication partner has already moved on to another topic. Sara's mom reports that these difficulties limit Sara's friendships. She reportedly will withdraw from a play situation if it becomes too dependent on language.

Sara's formalized testing consisted of the Goldman-Fristoe-Woodcock Test of Auditory Discrimination, which is designed to provide measures of speech-sound discrimination ability under ideal listening conditions plus a comparative measure of auditory discrimination in the presence of controlled background noise. Sara performed at the first percentile for both the quiet and noise subtest. A point to note was that Sara's posture changed with the noise subtest. She leaned forward and dropped her head as if trying to increase her ability to attend to the words being presented.

Following the testing, Sara eagerly explored the clinic environment. Her movement patterns were quick, which also matched her attention. There was also a sense of caution in her movement from one activity to the next that appeared to be related to her perception of space. Sara's mother also reported that Sara would frequently misunderstand words relating to space and movement.

Listening Program
After sharing some of the test results with Sara's mother, Sara was set up on a home program of Disc EASe for two 30-minute sessions. The body aspect most glaring at this point was her difficulty in orienting to her speech partner, reflected by her lack of presence during my interactions with her.

At the follow-up appointment three weeks later, Sara came bounding in, apprearing far more confident with herself. She exhibited a real presence that was not there initially. The Test of Auditory Discrimination was repeated with significant changes noted: she went from the first percentile to the 70th percentile for the quiet subtest and to the 84th percentile on the noise subtest. This time there was no shift in her posture for the noise subtest. It was truly easier for Sara.

Her mother reported that Sara has been responding faster to comments and questions, her speech is more fluent and she appears more willing to participate in conversations. She has also been more willing to try things out without having to observe them first. Expressing more emotion has also been new for Sara, including crying. Previously, she was a child who rarely cried or expressed how she was feeling.

Sara's program will be continually modified to continue to address the underlying difficulties contributing to her communication delays. The next step will be to address the underlying movement or body issues in a combined OT and speech treatment intensive.

Teacher Report
Name: Matt
6th grade
Molly Kaliher, Special Education Teacher

Documentated change with an adapted listening program for the classroom - provided by the Special Education Teacher.

Matt has struggled to read all through his academic career. His reading goal, as stated on his IEP dated October 1997, was to read 2.0 grade level material at a rate of 30 words per minute. At that time, a checklist was used daily to give Matt feedback about his reading session. A "great" day was when Matt read 20 words per minute with less than 6 errors. A "blah" day was when he read less than 15 words per minute with five or more errors.

Matt was identified as a LD student in first grade. I started working with him when he was in third grade. Methods used include: Direct Instruction Reading Mastery, Read Naturally and an assortment of trade books.

Matt began the Therapeutic Listening program on February 13, 1997. This was used in addition to his specially designed reading program. During the first 10 days, Matt did not complete reading activities. Instead, he worked on puzzles

and drawing activities. After the initial 10 days, a reading sample was taken (see graph below). Matt continued the integrated listening program for the remainder of the school year. He listened while he worked on reading activities.

Matt continued to listen at home during the summer months.

Significant events:
- Matt is able to read 4th grade level material.
- Matt perceives himself as a reader. He volunteered to read a passage at his 6th grade band concert.
- Matt has commented that he can finally "do things in 6th grade. I can read."
- Matt is attempting to participate in the regular 6th grade reading program.
- Prior to Therapeutic Listening, Matt accurately decoded the first word in a sentence 40% of the time. After listening, this improved to 90%.

Matt

	A	B	C	D
1	DATE	WPM	ERRORS	GRADE LEVEL
2	12/10/96	15	7	1.5
3	1/8/97	18	5	2.0
4	2/11/97	22	5	2.0
5	2/12/97	18	6	2.0
6	2/27/97	44	5	2.0
7	3/4/97	57	4	2.5
8	4/15/97	55	6	2.5
9	5/29/97	52	4	2.5
10	9/9/97	65	5	4.0
11	10/16/97	70	6	4.0
12	11/18/97	70	4	4.0
13	12/17/97	76	5	4.0
14	1/8/98	75	6	4.0

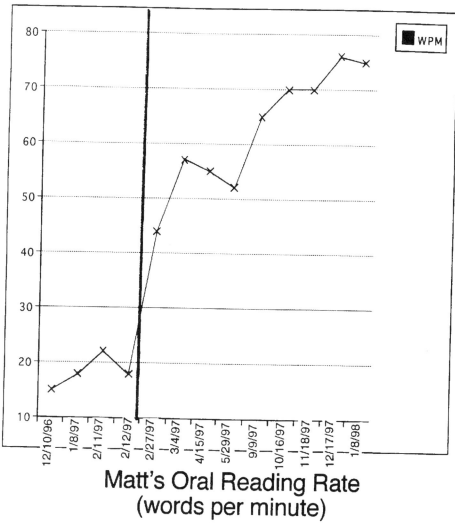

Matt's Oral Reading Rate
(words per minute)

Children's Drawings

Children's human figure drawings have been used as a part of assessment in occupational therapy as well as other disciplines. They reflect the developmental progression of a child's overall conceptual development, perceptually, intellectually, physically and emotionally. The stages and sequences of children's drawings are particularly uniform through time and space as well as across cultures and socioeconomic groups.

Occupational therapists in particular have been interested in children's drawings as graphic representations of a child's body scheme. Body scheme or precept requires a sensorimotor map of the body from which the child can move though space and motor plan. These maps are developed and refined though a child's physical interactions with the environment. Both motor planning and motor skill require a perception of how the body is put together and how it functions mechanically. The brain requires a sensory picture to move the body accurately. The more a child moves and the more variations of movement the child is able to perform, the more accurate the maps and the more able the child will be to navigate through space. Many of the drawings on the following pages demonstrate sometimes dramatic changes in body scheme and perceptual motor development as reflected in the rapid maturation of their self-portraits.

It is interesting to note that these drawings follow the consistent and reliable developmental progression of children's drawings throughout time, however, the time spans between the developmental stages is often abbreviated. Some of the children initially demonstrate severe delays in their drawings that are often quickly remedied with the addition of listening techniques into their sensory integrative programs.

The following is a brief synopsis of the developmental stages of children's drawings according to the exhaustive reseach of Joesph Di Leo M.D. recorded in his book, *Young Children and Their Drawings* (1970).

The kinesthetic stage spans from thirteen months to three years. This stage reflects the graphic movements; attention is on the 'how' versus 'what' is being drawn. The graphic movements have a predictable sequence that begins with a to and fro movement that is uninterrupted or a horizontal zigzag. Vertical, circular and skein like movements are more typically seen in the third year. As the child gains more cortical control over movement there is a transition between the kinesthetic and representational stage. This passage is never abrupt and often has frequent lapses into earlier levels with an upward and onward trend toward representational.

In the representational stage the child draws what he knows not what he sees. Initially the head is primary because of the child's focus on eating, speaking, seeing and hearing. The arms and legs emerge from the head since this is how the child is able to reach and move out into the world. At this point in time the body is ignored. The eyes are goggle like and are often the first facial feature to be drawn, followed by the mouth, nose and ears. The trunk appears around the age of five. The more mature trunk is longer than it is wide and larger than the head.

The final stage of human figure drawing is visual realism. At this point children draw what they see. In the transition between representational and visual realism, mixed profile and transparencies are often present. Brighter children often reach the final stage early, some as early as six years of age.

The following drawings have been collected from various therapists, parents and teachers around the country over the last several years. Not all the cases reflect the current guidelines for using Therapeutic Listening as they have evolved to achieve maximum effectiveness. Many of the following cases showing dramatic improvements emphasize the difficulty expressing actual abilities when sensory processing dysfunction interferes.

References

Harris, D. B., (1963). *Goodenough-harris drawing test*. San Antonio: The Pyschological Corporation, Harcourt Brace & Company.

Newton, M. & Thomson, M. E., (1976). *The Aston Index*. Wisbech, England: Learning Development Aids.

Di Leo, J., (1970). *Young children and their drawings*. New York: Brunner/Mozel, Inc.

Student: Jack
C.A.: 5.3 yrs

Denese Neigh, OTR, Tupper Lake, NY

Child with severe pervasive developmenal disorder; in-school program.

Significant History

♦ Third pregnancy, term with excessive maternal weight gain, detached placenta, confined to bed last 4 months.

♦ Vaginal delivery, head presentation, initial Apgar 9, birth weight 10 pounds, 1 ounce.

♦ Unable to breast feed.

♦ Possible early lead exposure.

♦ One older brother is identified as LD.

♦ Biological father was physically abusive and eventually left the family. Restraining order was necessary during the first 12 months of his placement with us secondary to continued threats of "taking Jack away from mom."

♦ History is negative for ear infections, but early history is sketchy with the family under a great deal of stress and moving often.

♦ Speech was significantly delayed with referral to programming for the deaf following initial audiogram. Subsequent audiograms revealed hearing to be within normal limits.

♦ By age 4.8 years, Jack had been placed with 9 different child care providers due to his lack of personal safety skills.

♦ Jack did not interact with other children, nor would they with him; he was highly distractible and impulsive.

♦ Speech described as rapid, loud, echolalic, repetitive and marked by neologisms.

♦ He resisted verbal prompts.

♦ Recommendations included psychological testing, medical consultation and speech language services due to "potential for development of some expressive language skills" given his advanced expressive language scores on the *Goldman Fristoe Test of Articulation*.

♦ Jack was referred to our program (last resort) in spring of '98 (5.3 years) and I evaluated him on 5/4/98. At that time, two-person physical intervention was necessary to ensure his safety and the safety of others.

Assessment (see scores with drawings)

Jack was very active but able to respond to directives accompanied by gesture and physical contact (placing my hand on his forearm). He withdrew from all physical contact that was not within his visual field. Eye contact was fleeting. Oral motor concerns were monumental: Jack refused most foods and smelled or touched food first; he presented food at sides of mouth only, followed by limited mastication, no rotary chewing and washed all food down with large amounts of milk. Pocketing large amounts of unchewed food was an ongoing safety and nutritional issue. Often subtle, but persistent visual self-stimulation was noted. He wanted to stand at the easel and paint but would then place large drops of paint (3 colors only) at the top of the paper and let them drip down. Hand flapping appeared when Jack was agitated or excited. Speech was bizarre with fragmented and convoluted sentence structure. His neologisms were very creative. Enuresis occurred nightly.

Jack liked percussive music activities, immediately learning patterns with accurate commitment to long-term memory. He preferred the computer to toys, could not ride a bike, had poor balance and appeared to have no idea how to use playground equipment. Eye and hand dominance were not established (nor is hand now). Jack could not localize to sound and demonstrated behaviors consistent with hyperacuisis.

Note

I knew immediately that Jack's visual perceptual and auditory skills were great strengths, as well as sources of frustration. I believed that those heightened skills combined with the poor praxis, a challenging home life and probable superior cognitive abilities (psych said he was borderline MR with splinter skills) had created a time bomb. Because of his size and age (he was placed in preschool), we didn't have much time.

Listening Program

We started with EASe I twice a day during the last couple of weeks of summer school, primarily in a little play tent in the hall with lots of tactile and oral motor toys. All sessions were 20 minutes, 2X a day for five days. On June 10th we added five minutes of ST 101. The family could not handle a home program. Jack was initially hesitant about the headphones but tolerated them, seeming to sense they could offer something he needed. Though we negotiated whose turn it was to listen (mine or his) and which CD to choose (choice of two), listening was not optional and Jack respected that right from the beginning.

Initial Changes

♦ Enuresis stopped.

♦ Increased eye contact.

♦ Behaviors decreased with fewer trips to the padded time out room (charted data)

♦ Beginning to turn his head in direction of the speaker in response to his name spoken at a conversational level. These changes had occurred by the end of the two available treatment weeks and were still solidly in place when school resumed in September.

Follow-up

Jack entered the program again in September, resuming treatment late September. Therapy was one on one in a large gym. I set up large motor activities and used a fanny pack and headset. I also used lots of oral motor toys. We ended sessions with prewriting and manipulative on the floor. I used wedges, beanbag chairs and bolsters on the floor for these tasks.

Follow-up Program

Treatment was still twice daily using EASe 1 and 2 and ST 101. He called it the "fire music." December 1, '98, I reduced sessions to one approximately two to three times weekly. he was transitioning to kindergarten and doing well.

Changes continued to be dramatic and we began transitioning Jack into a regular kindergarten (onsite) immediately, with support of a 1 to 1 staff person. He was amazing. He participated in the Christmas kindergarten play; not only with a speaking part but serving as a prompter for the other kids, having learned all of their lines, as well as his own. Jack has a very sophisticated and slightly skewed sense of humor. His peers liked him but didn't quite know what to make of him, however, they were more adept than their teacher. She had a large class and simply didn't know what to do with him. In a moment of extreme frustration and revelation (to me), she said, "Listen, I just want to get him through a game of Duck-Duck-Goose. That's what I care about." Jack quickly surpassed his peers in reading, math, art and music, while challenges to learning decreased and behaviors began to increase. Jack's social skills remained weaker than the adults could accept. We utilized social scripting and Therapeutic Listening was implemented on an as-needed basis, with Jack often requesting "his music."

It was time to reevaluate in March of '99 (please see attached scores) and to go to committee again. I got the placement tabled once more, but by that time they had had enough of me. When the final meeting was scheduled, I wasn't invited and Jack was placed in a contained classroom. It is a 6 to 1 plus 1 special classroom for ED kids, with inclusion in regular classes as appropriate. I am unable to treat him as the district has their own therapists and they are not Therapeutic Listening trained, and, despite my efforts, don't express an interest. Jack is doing okay overall and is taught at a pace consistent with his learning style and abilities. I do see an autistic child from another district in Jack's class daily, so am able to keep track of his progress. When he has a behavioral episode, his teacher, a believer, will express her frustration at not having access to this treatment, not just for Jack, but for all of her kids.

I was very fortunate to have encountered Jack immediately after my initial Therapeutic Listening course. He's a great kid: smart, funny,

---

a real Jim Carrey kind of guy, who I suspect is a real genius, too. I hope I gave Jack the skills to identify his needs and to be able to advocate for himself regarding them. To me, that is also a big part of what we have to do for kids like Jack.

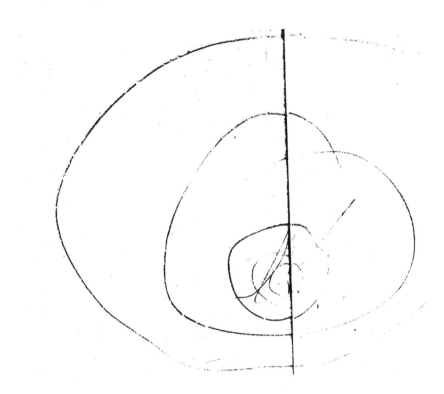

Kinesthetic stage around age two. Drawn on two large sheets of paper. Very poor fine motor control.

Date: 5-04-98; CA: 5yrs, 3 mos.
Initial drawing

Initial scores:
Peabody:
Gross motor: 36 mos
Fine motor: 50 mos
AE: 48 mo (mean motor age equivelent)

TVMS: Score=60 mo

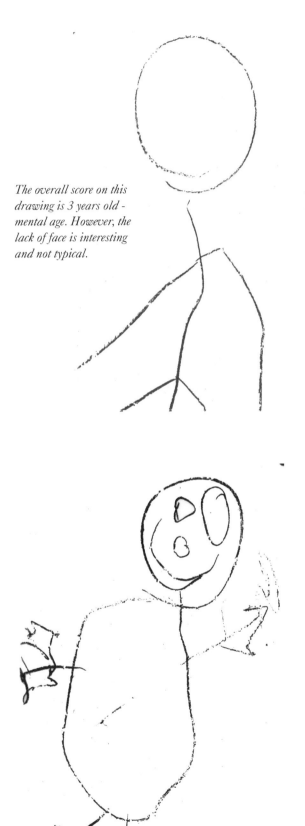

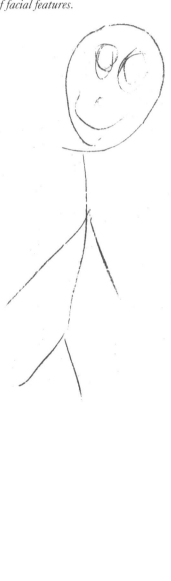

The overall score on this drawing is 3 years old - mental age. However, the lack of face is interesting and not typical.

Mental age : 5 years old. Goggle-like eyes typical of 1st appearance of facial features.

5.5 years old - mental age. The appearance of the trunk typically is seen in 5 year old's drawings.

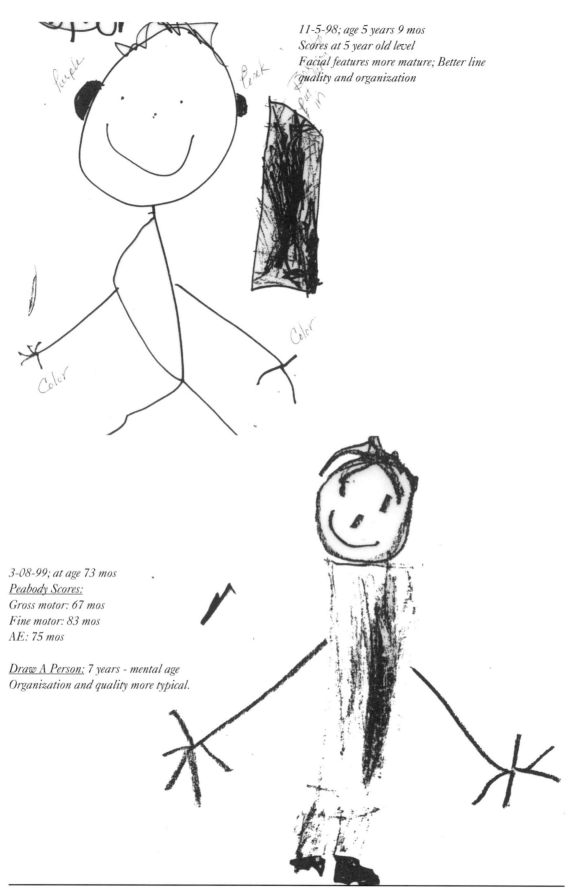

11-5-98; age 5 years 9 mos
Scores at 5 year old level
Facial features more mature; Better line
quality and organization

Purple

Penk

Color

Color

3-08-99; at age 73 mos
Peabody Scores:
Gross motor: 67 mos
Fine motor: 83 mos
AE: 75 mos

Draw A Person: 7 years - mental age
Organization and quality more typical.

Name: Mitchell
CA: 5 yrs 6 mo

Denese Neigh, OTR, Tupper Lake, NY

Child with moderate sensory defensiveness. In school program with follow-up home program.

Significant History

- Mitchell is the product of a normal birth and delivery. He was described as a colicky baby.
- He has a significant history for middle ear infections beginning at 4 months that were treated with antibiotics.
- Due to continued infections he had PE tubes placed at 14 months and then again at 18 months.
- His mother described him as clumsy and accident-prone.

Assessment (see scores with drawings)

Mitchell demonstrated moderate sensory defensiveness. Sensory history revealed olfactory sensitivities to people, perfumes, food odors and cat litter. He presents with a hyperactive gag reflex. He avoids physical contact with peers. He presents with auditory defensiveness, he states that certain sounds hurt his ears. He was unable to attend music class and physical education due to noise levels. He grinds his teeth during sleep and has occasional enuresis. He does not receive speech service since the evaluation findings indicated a central auditory processing disorder for which there is no treatment.

His teacher referred Mitchell to occupational therapy. The referral concerns were due to his difficulties participating in music and gym class. Initial evaluation showed delays in gross, fine and visual motor skills.

Listening Program
Direct therapy was provided for 30 minutes 5 times a week. His OT sessions were conducted in the classroom during snack and free play. Mitchell would initiate his listening to Mozart for Modulation-Modified while he was having his snack. This was followed by use of gross motor equipment that included a Lycra swing. SAMONAS CDs of Classic ST 101 and Chamber ST 104 were added to this 30- minute listening sessions. His initial treatment session lasted for 4 weeks followed by a two-week spring break. During this break there was some sporadic follow-through by his family. Upon his return to school 4 more weeks of treatment were completed prior to re-evaluation and resultant discharge from OT due to dramatic improvements and resolution of the referral concerns.

Initial Change

Improvements include the ability to participate in physical education and music class and an increase in social skills as evidenced by his newfound ability to make friends. His mother reported that he was invited to a birthday party for the first time. Others noted that he was much more relaxed and happy.

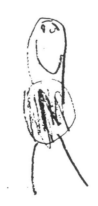

1/21/99 CA: 66 mo

PEABODY DMS:
Gross Motor: 49 mo,
Fine Motor: 50 mo
VMI: 21 percentile
Visual: 99th percentile

Draw A Person:
Mental age: 4 years

Mitchell 12345678

4/21/99 CA: 69 mo
PEABODY DMS:
Gross Motor: 71 mos
Fine Motor: 72 mos
VMI: 73 percentile Visual: 99.2 percentile
(Please refer to Draw A Person samples.)

Draw A Person Mental age: 5 years

Discharged from direct OT services;
all referral concerns resolved.

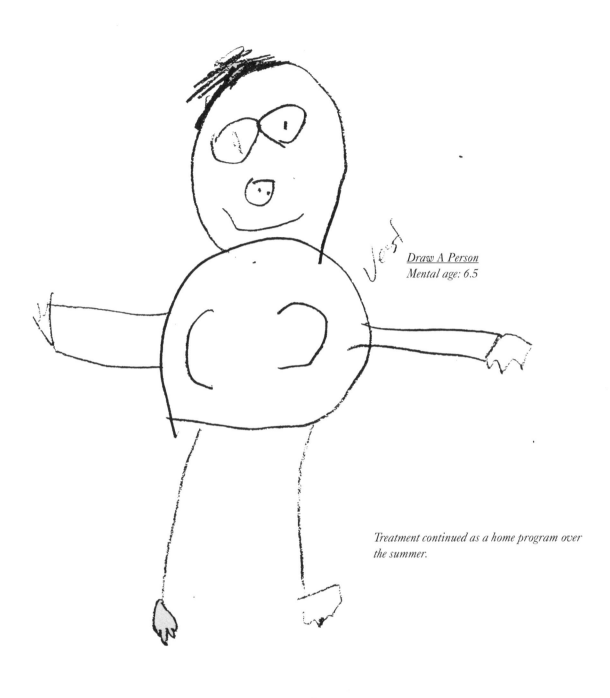

Draw A Person
Mental age: 6.5

Treatment continued as a home program over the summer.

Mitchell   6/8/99

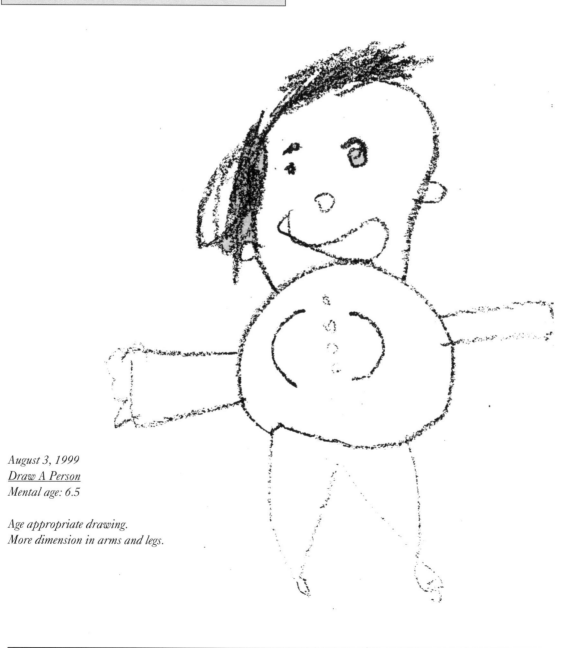

August 3, 1999
Draw A Person
Mental age: 6.5

Age appropriate drawing.
More dimension in arms and legs.

Name: Dave
Age: 6.2

Ginger Mitchell, Wheat Ridge, CO.

Modulated music home program intervention for a child with moderate sensory defensiveness and sensory integrative dysfunction.

Dave first came for a Therapeutic Listening consult on 7/20/99. (The first drawing was done at this time.) The issues at that time were his frequent melt downs, delayed fine motor skills, auditory defensiveness, difficulties with attention and following directions. He started on EASe 3 for 30 minutes twice daily.

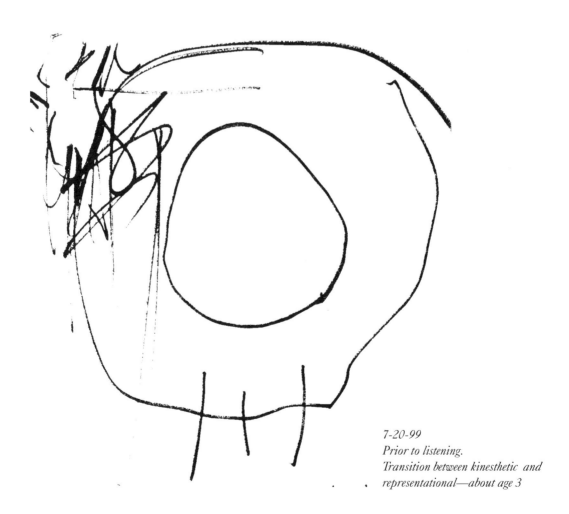

7-20-99
Prior to listening.
Transition between kinesthetic and
representational—about age 3

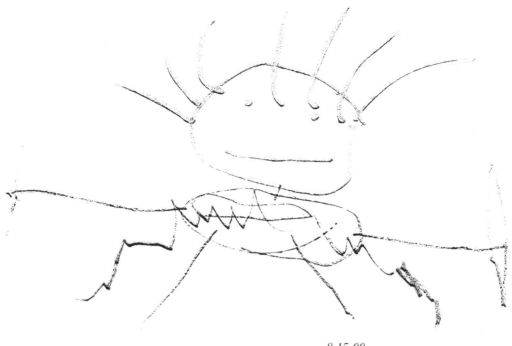

8-15-99
MA: 5 years

He was seen again on 8/15/99. Mom reported an initial increase in temper tantrums which subsided and decreased significantly. Dave continued to improve with respect to attention and fine motor skills. His interest in fine motor exploration was exhibited by requesting to draw and play with blocks. He was eating better and others reported that his behavior was more mature.

MA: 5.5
Better organization; head and trunk more proportionate.
9-20-99

Name: Kiani
Age: 5 years 11 months

Ginger Mitchell, Wheat Ridge, CO.

Home listening program with in-clinic occupational therapy and speech/language therapy.

Kiani was seen for OT from the age of 4 when she had significant difficulties with somatosensory and spatial processing. She had significant difficulties with fine and gross motor praxis skills. She also had moderate to severe tactile and auditory defensiveness. She had OT twice a week for about 6 months and once a week since then. She also had speech therapy once a week for two and half years for articulation and word finding problems. Although Kiani made progress in each of these, it was slow.

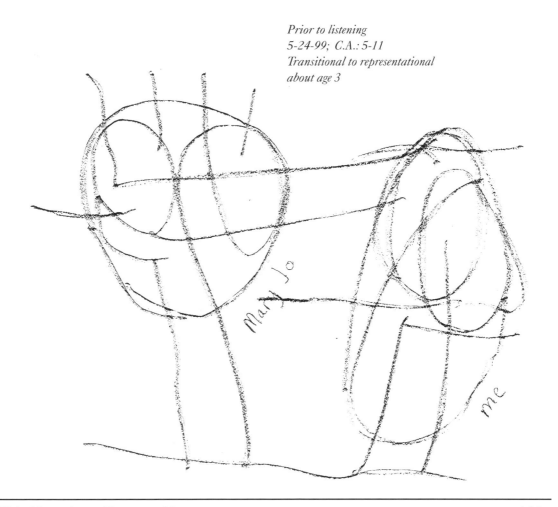

Prior to listening
5-24-99; C.A.: 5-11
Transitional to representational
about age 3

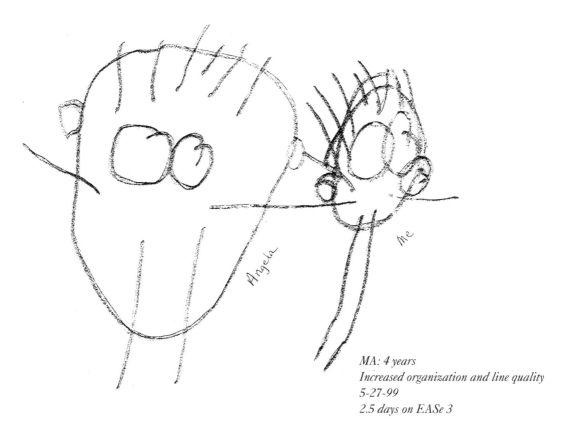

MA: 4 years
Increased organization and line quality
5-27-99
2.5 days on EASe 3

Kiani continued on this program for about 2 months and continued to have improvement in decreasing the number of temper tantrums, increased tolerance to clothes and to being touched. Her balance improved dramatically, as did her willingness to try new things. She learned to ride a 2-wheel bike and jump rope. Also, she was able to play outside without being overly bothered by the noise of traffic.

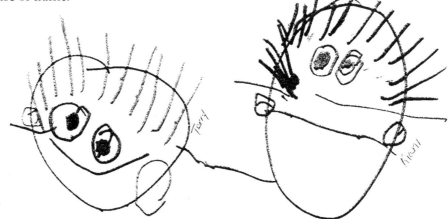

6-11-99
after 2.5 weeks EASe 3
MA: 4 years
Improved detail in the face. The addition of pupils.
Increased line quality.

Name: Nicky
Age: 5

Lori Rothman, OTR, New York, NY

Gifted child with mild
modulation problems.

Drawings done by a gifted five year old with mild sensory modulation difficulties after listening to 10 minutes of ST Classic while waiting for his sibling who was receiving direct therapy services.

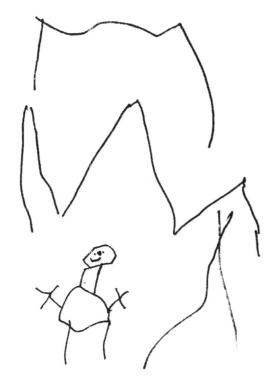

Prior to listening
MA: 5

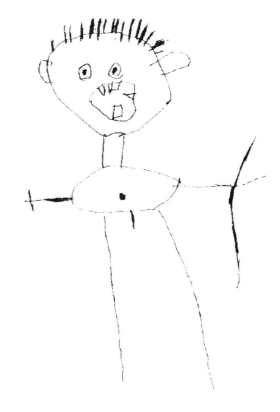

MA: 6
More detail reflective of increased focus and improved attention. Able to express actual potential.

Name: Jared
7 year old, 2nd grader

Joanne Holmes, OTR, St. Petersburg, FL

In-school listening program.

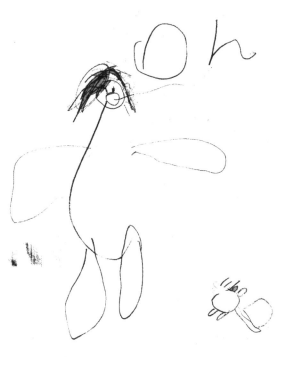

(Left) 1-29-01 Drawings prior to listening. Child with attention and learning issues.
MA: 5
Began listening today to EASe and Baroque, 2X 30 minutes; 5 days/week.

(Below) 2 weeks into _school_ listening program; Baroque—Modified, EASe 2/day for 30 minutes. Teacher noticed more focus during class time.
Score-MA: 5

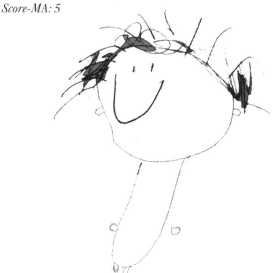

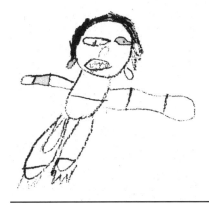

2-29-01 MA: 7 years
Addition of Carulli to program in a ST level.

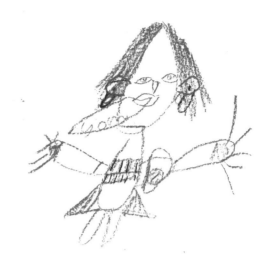

4-01
MA: 8 years
Increase in detail about the face and body.

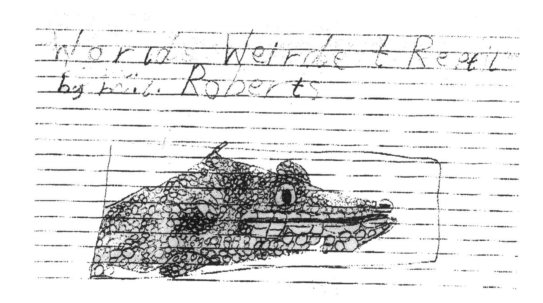

4-22-01
Listening program included Baroque, EASe 1 (2X30
minutes alternating) and Carulli in ST format. Initiated
at school and then home follow-up midway through the
program.

Name: Andrew
Age: 6.2

Genevieve Jereb, OTR, Madison, WI

Child with mild cerebral palsy.

Andrew listened to EASe 1 2X/day for the time period 7-10 to 7-22-00. The drawings that follow are his progression in grapho-motor skill. On 7-21 he requested paper and drew for 30 minutes. This was the first time in his life that he initiated drawing. Mom noted that he drew actual pictures without prompting. By the end of July his pencil grip was less palmar and more of a tripod grasp (this was the first change in grasp in a year). He also dressed himself independently for the first time.

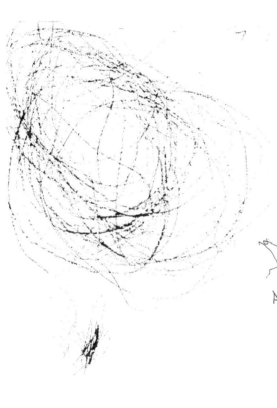

7-10-00 Initial listening assessment identified difficulties with sensory modulation.

Score: 2 years
Typical of kinesthetic stage.

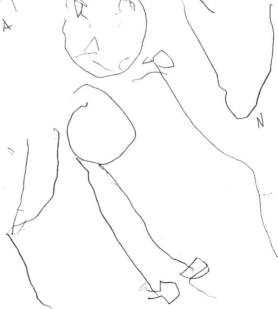

7-20-00
Continues with EASe. Mom reports restlessness at bedtime, much more emotional expression, not accepting 'no', whining and tantrums. Requesting drawing for the first time ever. First time pictures are not just scribbles.

Score - MA: 4 years

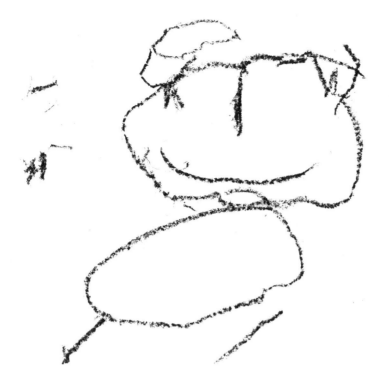

7-21-00
Tantrums and whining decreased but still present. Switching hands while drawing. Pictures are more organized with some correct spatial components.

Score MA: 4.2

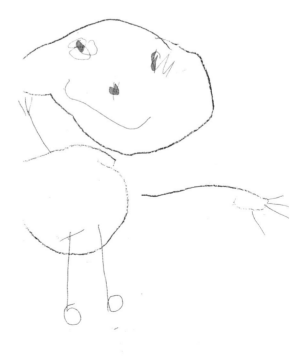

7-22-00 Picture of Mom

Drew spontaneously. Darker crayon pressure; more face details correctly placed and smiling. He's *never* just drawn a picture, previously just scribbled. Arms attached, body grounded. He is also staying focused for longer periods. Has dressed himself independently for the first time.

Score MA: 5 years

My Dog Skip

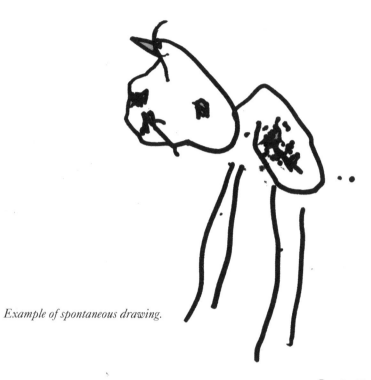

Example of spontaneous drawing.

7-22-00

Name: Jennifer
Age: 4 years

Home listening
program/sensory diet – see full
case report on page 4-13.

3-09-01
VMI - 3.9
Drawing at 3 year transitional level.

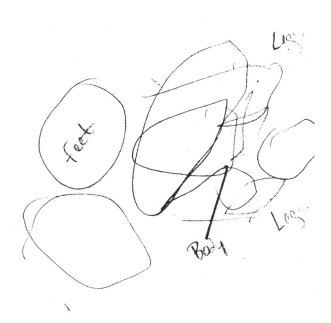

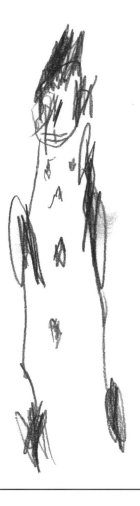

7/10/01 after listening to EASe and CQ Carulli
CA: 4.4
VMI: 4-2
Drawing Score MA: 4 years

Name: Maria
Age: 4.9

Maria has severe sensory processing difficulties especially in visual and vestibular processing areas. Her Therapeutic Listening program included EASe 1, Baroque—Modified, Carulli-ST and Sounds of Nature.

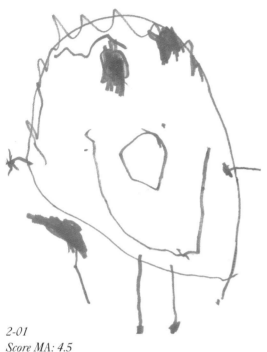

2-01
Score MA: 4.5

5-01; CA: 5.0
Following a varied listening program: EASe 1, Baroque–Modified, Carulli, Sounds of Nature.

Score MA: 6 years
Arms and legs present and proportionate. Head in proportion to trunk. Her parents noted a marked increase in self-regulation, speech/language development and comfort, safety and judgement issues out in the community.

I see **Maria** looking at me!

Name: Frederick
Age: 5

Home listening program
with a sensory diet
consisting of heavy work.

Intellectually gifted five year old boy with severe sensory modulation difficulties and autistic like behaviors. Very impulsive, difficult to maintain in preschool environment. Started listening to EASe 1. Dawing at 5 years mental age.

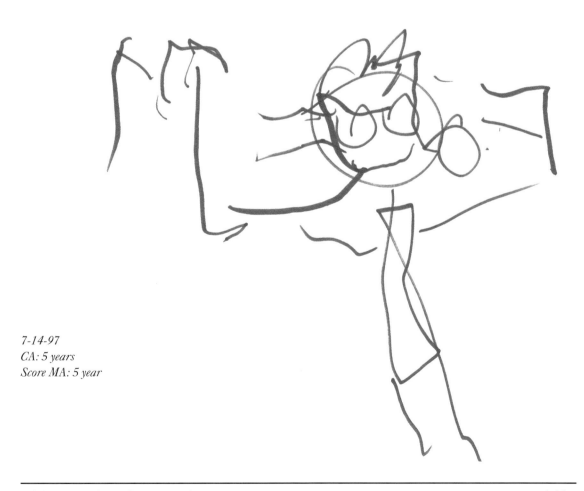

7-14-97
CA: 5 years
Score MA: 5 year

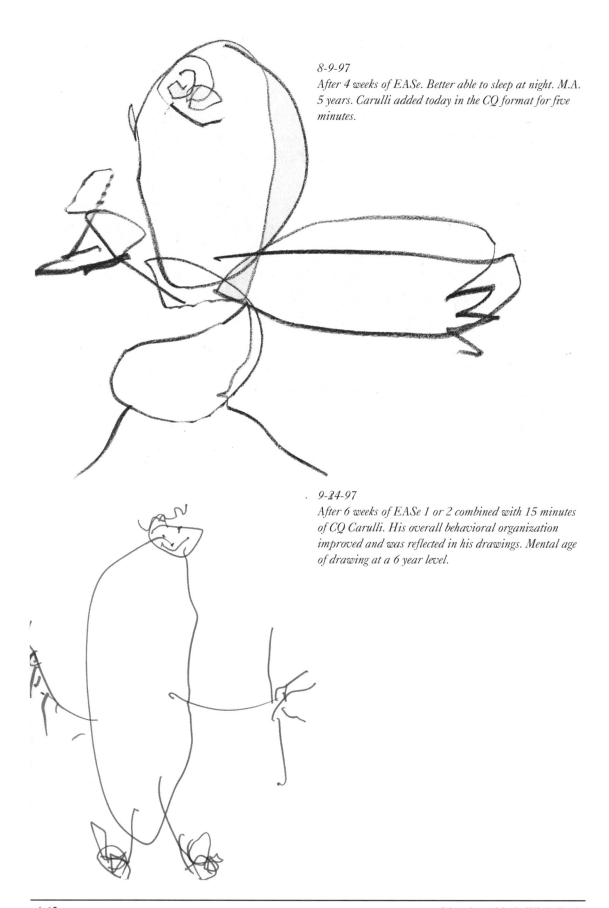

8-9-97
*After 4 weeks of EASe. Better able to sleep at night. M.A.
5 years. Carulli added today in the CQ format for five
minutes.*

9-24-97
*After 6 weeks of EASe 1 or 2 combined with 15 minutes
of CQ Carulli. His overall behavioral organization
improved and was reflected in his drawings. Mental age
of drawing at a 6 year level.*

Name: Michael
Age: 9.9

Linda Lutzeier, MOT, OTR, Ann Arbor, MI

Listening program initiated at school; followed up at home after a short period.

Michael was eligible for special education services as Emotionally Impaired and Speech and Language Impaired. He was referred for an occupational therapy evaluation at the end of fourth grade due to concerns related to writing and sensory processing. He also had difficulties with reading, math and spelling.

The Wilbarger Touch Pressure Protocol was implemented, a sensory diet of heavy work activities was developed and Michael was introduced to Therapeutic Listening to address identified difficulties with auditory defensiveness, bilateral coordination, laterality, visual motor integration and markedly delayed self drawings. Michael listened to 30 minutes of EASe 1 and 7 minutes of Carulli (CQ level).

5/97
Draw A Person prior to listening program.
Score MA: 3.6

VMI Score: 5th percentile
AE: 6.2

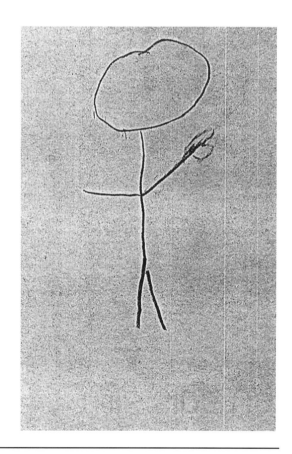

7-10-97
After two sessions 30 minutes of EASe 1 and 7 minutes of
Carulli, a week apart.

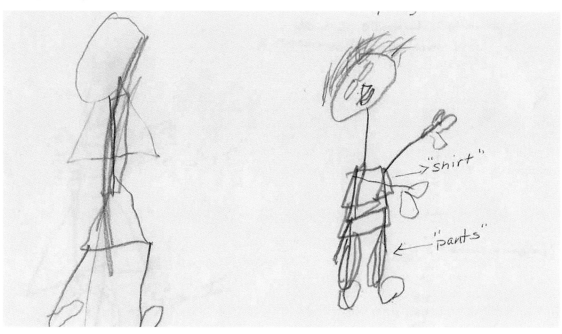

7-17-97
After three sessions of 30 minutes of EASe 1 and 7
minutes of Carulli, a week apart.
MA: 7 years, three months

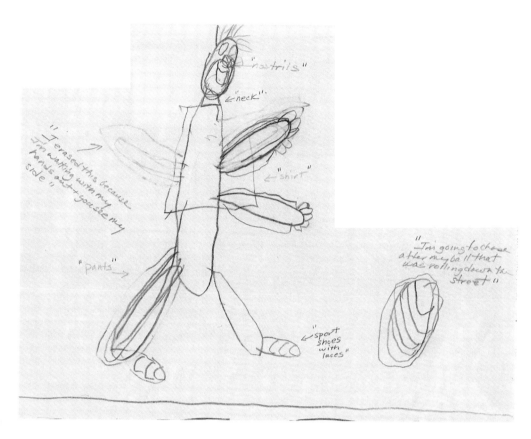

"nostrils"

←"neck"

"I erased this because I'm waiting with my hands out + you see my side"

←"shirt"

"I'm going to chase after my ball that was rolling down the street"

"pants"→

←"sport shoes with laces"

7-24-97
MA: 8.0

Michael continued to listen 3 out of seven days a week until 8-21-97 when he was retested. VMI score: 15 percentile; AE: 7.0

Name: Demiko
Age: 6.10

Linda Lutzeier, MOT, OTR, Ann Arbor, MI

In-school listening program.

Demiko was determined eligible for special education services on 1/99 as Educable Mentally Impaired, with additional concerns related to increased activity such as drumming on his desk, spinning and sliding along the floor, as well as poor focused attention to most school activity. He was moved to a self-contained classroom. During his OT sessions, he worked on fine motor activities in the classroom and listened to Carulli CQ level or Romantic CQ level, 15-20 minutes, one time per week, for 6 weeks. There was marked improvement in focused attention and eagerness to write and draw throughout the week, even when the OT was not present, and he was not listening to the therapeutic music.

3-5-99
Score MA: 4.3

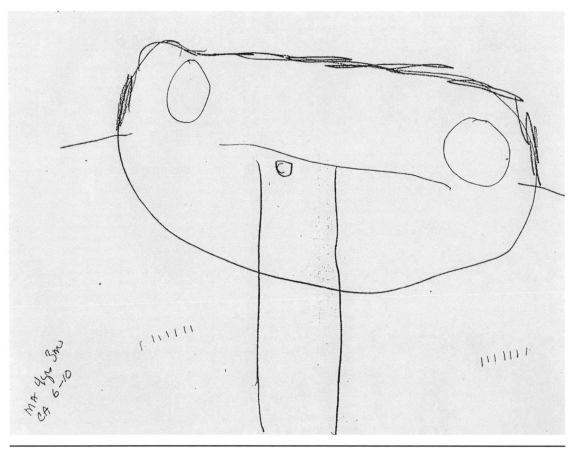

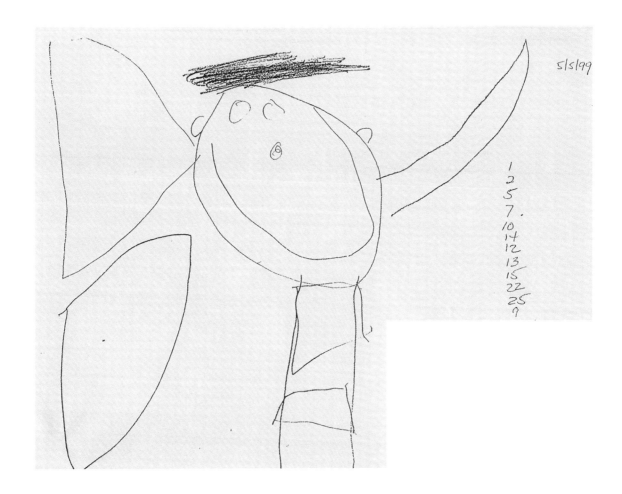

Alex was labled Learning Disabled with a long history of sensory defensiveness. He had had auditory, tactile and visual defensiveness. As a very young child, he was easily overwhelmed and would slip into a trance-like state to cope with sensory overload. His defensiveness was treated with the Wilbarger Protocol and a sensory diet with heavy work activities that lessened his tactile defensiveness. His gross motor skills improved significantly; however, he continued to struggle with fine motor skills, weak organization skills and poor written expression. He had no interest in drawing. His DAP was 5 years, 9 months prior to having Therapeutic Listening added to his weekly OT sessions.

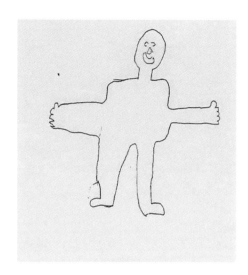

He listened to Carulli CQ level for 10-20 minutes for 8 sessions.

His DAP improved to 7 years, 9 months (this represents a 2 year improvement in 2 months, listening only one time per week). His mother reported a sudden interest in drawing at home and while waiting for meals in restaurants.

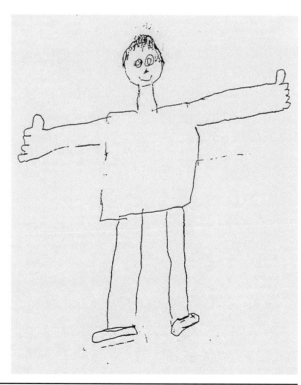

Name: Ian
Age: 8.7

Linda Lutzeier, MOT, OTR, Ann Arbor, MI

In-school listening program.

Ian was a third grade student in a general education classroom. He has a diagnosis of neurofibromatosis and is eligible for special education as Learning Disabled. He also had significant problems with attention and regulating activity level. He was in constant motion in the classroom and was constantly throwing himself to the floor, rocking in his chair and bumping into the furniture.

11-12-98
CA: 8.7
Score MA: 6.1

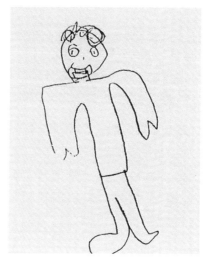

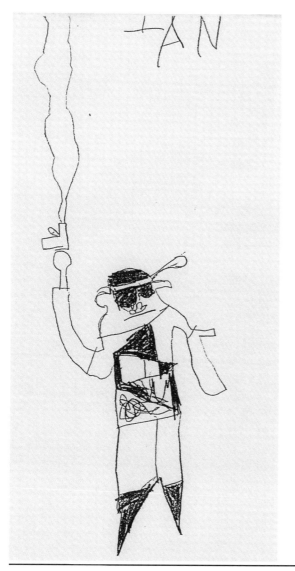

1-7-98
CA: 8.9
Score MA: 8.3
Listened once per week in the classroom to EASe 1 1 and CQ levels of Carulli and/or Romantic. Listening times ranged from 15-25 minutes.

Labeled 'severly emotionally
disturbed;' placed in
self-contained classroom.
In-school listening program.

Writing sample prior to listening

(92)

3-9-98

D.O.L. ? Saw
Betty and
Ioa on Hallow-1.
I am angry.

Watch your handwriting.

Jerrys book fell down.
My sister likes
pretty cp+s.

6 Th man drew drew a map
for Ars town.
2 My parents and I
found a fluffy kitten.
1. Dear Sally,
I haven't any gum
to give you.
2 Your friend, Betty.

I dun

Charles had been put on a strict behavior management program and was described by those who knew him as being a very angry kid. As an OT it was clear to me that sensory defensiveness was an issue. I placed Charles on a Disc EASe 1 Therapeutic Listening program for 30 minutes twice daily. The first two weeks were like a roller coaster ride, and aggressive outbursts were frequent. Just as we considered reducing his listening time, something shifted for Charles. All aggression subsided. Academic performance took a leap. After 4 weeks, I compared a writing sample from his journal with his initial writing sample. The comparison was astonishing. Changes in spatial organization were dramatic. His teacher informed me that Charles looked happy.

Writing sample 4-15-98

5-15-98

I won't go with you.
Has she gone to the lake for
summer vacation?